Audiology & Communication Disorders

An Overview

Audiology & Communication Disorders

An Overview

LARRY E. HUMES, PhD

Professor
Department of Speech and Hearing Sciences
Indiana University
Bloomington, Indiana

FRED H. BESS, PhD

Professor and Chair
Department of Hearing and Speech Sciences
Vanderbilt Bill Wilkerson Center for Otolaryngology
and Communication Sciences
Vanderbilt University Medical Center
Nashville, Tennessee

 Wolters Kluwer | Lippincott Williams & Wilkins
Health

Philadelphia • Baltimore • New York • London
Buenos Aires • Hong Kong • Sydney • Tokyo

Acquisitions Editor: Peter Sabatini
Managing Editor: Kevin C. Dietz
Marketing Manager: Allison Noplock
Artist: Jonathan Dimes
Designer: Candice Carta-Myers
Compositor: Aptara
Printer: RR Donnelley-China

Library of Congress Cataloging-in-Publication Data

Humes, Larry.
   Audiology and communication disorders : an overview /
Larry E. Humes, Fred H. Bess.
      p. ; cm.
   Includes bibliographical references and index.
   ISBN-13: 978-0-7817-7555-7 (soft : alk. paper)
   ISBN-10: 0-7817-7555-8 (soft : alk. paper) 1. Audiology. 2. Hearing. 3. Hearing disorders.
4. Communicative disorders. I. Bess, Fred H. II. Title.
   [DNLM: 1. Hearing—physiology. 2. Hearing Disorders.
3. Communication Disorders. 4. Hearing Impaired Persons—rehabilitation.
WV 270 H922a 2009]
   RF290.H86 2009
   617.8—dc22

                                            2007046532

10 9 8 7 6 5 4 3 2 1

To our wives, Susie and Marty
Our children, Danny, Amy, Rick, Andy, Liz, Lauren, and Adam
Our grandchildren, Matthew, Molly, Jack, and Noah
and
To the undergraduate and graduate students with whom
we have had the pleasure to work
over the past few decades

Table of Contents

Preface

We have co-authored an introductory textbook in audiology, *Audiology: The Fundamentals*, that will be in its fourth edition at the time of this writing. When each revision of this text would go out for review, the reviews were very informative and frequently split down the middle, with half wanting less depth and breadth of coverage and the other half wanting more depth and breadth. Obviously, it is not possible to meet the needs of both groups.

It was also apparent that the assumed target audience differed between the two groups of reviewers. Those desiring a more elementary treatment envisioned future speech-language pathologists, or more broadly future "nonaudiologists," as the target group. On the other hand, those reviewers who desired more advanced treatment were using the text in classes designed for audiologists, either at the upper undergraduate level or during the initial year of graduate or professional programs.

So, in prior revisions of that text, we tried to work out a compromise, such as moving material to "advanced supplements" at the end of each chapter. When split feedback from reviewers was received yet again as we were preparing for the fourth edition of *Fundamentals*, we spoke with the publisher about the possibility of simply developing two books: one at a more elementary level that would meet the needs of one group of reviewers and one at a more advanced level that would meet the needs of the other group. The publisher agreed with this approach and the fourth edition of the *Fundamentals* text represents the more advanced treatment of audiology. This text, on the other hand, represents the more elementary treatment of the material and is set in a broader speech-communication context.

ORGANIZATION

This book is divided into three main sections. In the first section, Chapters 1 to 3, a very broad overview of the "normal" or typical human communication is provided. This overview is framed around the "communication chain," an extension of the "speech chain" popularized many years ago by Denes & Pinson (1963; 1994). The communication chain is used to demonstrate the central role that hearing plays in everyday communication and in its development. This helps one to better understand the impact of hearing loss experienced at different ages on the development of the communication chain.

After demonstrating the critical importance of sound and hearing to communication (especially spoken communication) in the first section, the next section of the text (Chapters 4 to 6) is devoted to the description of various disorders that result in hearing loss and the impact of this hearing loss on communication. The point is made that it is important to identify hearing loss as early as possible to minimize its negative impact on communication. Because this text is primarily directed toward those planning to be in professions other than audiology, the focus is placed on screening procedures for the detection of hearing loss, rather than procedures for detailed diagnostic procedures. However, it is still likely that such professionals will need to understand audiological information for the children and adults with whom they will be working. As a result, information on the interpretation of basic diagnostic measures, including pure-tone audiometry, speech audiometry, and immittance measurements, is also presented in this section.

The final section of this book (Chapters 7 and 8) discusses approaches to the treatment of hearing loss once it has been identified. Here, it is assumed that the child or adult with impaired hearing is a part of the hearing world (as opposed to the Deaf world) and wishes to remain a part of "hearing culture." As such, the main treatment alternatives are hearing aids and cochlear implants, depending primarily on the severity of the hearing loss. Again, the assumption is that the reader of this text will not likely become an audiologist in the future, but will be interacting with adults and children with impaired hearing who have been seen by an audiologist. As a result, the focus will not be on the procedural details of selecting, fitting, and evaluating hearing aids or cochlear implants on patients, but on understanding the processes and the results from these processes to better manage the hearing-impaired person's communication.

FEATURES

This text makes use of several pedagogical features to enhance learning. Each chapter, for example, begins with a set of chapter objectives and concludes with a brief summary. Chapter review questions are at the end of each chapter to facilitate integration of the material. Five different types of vignettes—Experiments, Conceptual Demos, Further Discussion, Clinical Applications, and Historical Notes—are used throughout the text to drive home key points or to elaborate on them to facilitate understanding. In addition, Key Terms are identified at the beginning of each chapter, then highlighted and defined at first use in that chapter. These, and other terms, are defined as well in the Glossary at the end of the text.

ANCILLARIES

The CD-ROM that accompanies this text provides a wealth of interactive activities to reinforce understanding, including:

#1A

- A glossary with audio pronunciation
- Interactive screening tests
- Labeling exercises to reinforce terms and concepts from the text
- Chapter quizzes
- Case studies
- Animations of the anatomical structures
- Audio and video demonstrations (these are marked in the margins with audio or video icons to direct the reader to the accompanying CD. Additional details indicate exactly which clip coincides with the icon.)

For instructors, there are PowerPoint slides for each chapter and an Instructor's test generator to help teach the course more effectively.

We hope that this text meets the needs of those teaching undergraduates in need of a broad understanding of audiology, but who do not envision themselves to be "future audiologists." Perhaps, with this text and some luck, we'll be able to change the minds of at least some of them!

LARRY E. HUMES, PHD
FRED H. BESS, PHD

Reviewers

Jeff Brockett
Assistant Professor
Communication Sciences and Disorders
Idaho State University
Pocatello, ID

Bob Oyler
Professor & Chair
Mississippi University for Women
Dept. of Speech-Language Pathology
Columbus, MS

Lori Pakulski
Associate Professor
Health & Rehab Services
University of Toledo
Toledo, OH

Cynthia Richburg
Associate Professor
Special Education and Clinical Services
Indiana University of Pennsylvania
Indiana, PA

CHAPTER 1

The Communication Chain

CHAPTER OBJECTIVES

- To understand the basic components of the communication chain as the framework that facilitates the exchange of information, ideas, and emotions between two human beings;
- To identify key benchmarks in the typical development of the communication chain; and
- To appreciate the potential consequences of breaks in the communication brought about by impaired hearing.

KEY TERMS AND DEFINITIONS

- **Communication chain:** The chain of events that is initiated by a person (the talker or sender) who wishes to share information, ideas, or emotions with another person (the listener or receiver). In typical auditory-oral communication, this begins with the talker's conceptualization of the information or ideas to be exchanged and the initiation of speech production, which sends an acoustic signal to the listener. The listener's auditory system converts the arriving acoustical information to neural signals; these neural signals are processed by the listener's brain to decipher the speaker's message.
- **Language:** The code used by members of the same culture or group to decipher or produce sequences of sounds capable of communicating thoughts, ideas, and actions to other members of the same culture or group. Two key components are the lexicon (mental dictionary), which matches sound sequences to objects or actions, and syntax (grammar), which contains the rules by which words are sequenced in a language to form meaningful phrases and sentences.
- **Hearing impairment:** A loss of hearing that results in a need to have sounds increased in intensity, to levels greater than that normally heard by young adults, so as to be heard by the individual. The need for greater intensity to hear the sound is typically due to a disorder of some type located in the auditory system somewhere between the outer ear and the auditory portions of the brain.

It has been argued that communication of abstract concepts, thoughts, and ideas is a truly unique human experience, part of what distinguishes humans from other animals. This is not limited to communication about complex ideas or notions such as philosophical, religious, or political viewpoints, but includes many everyday aspects of communication as well. For example, consider the following simple scenario. You are planning a trip with a friend in which a map is consulted and costs are estimated for travel and accommodations—a very "concrete" exchange. Yet, this simple everyday dialogue between two friends involves the use and exchange of considerable abstract information. In this example, the exchange might include the processing of visual information on a map, perhaps a small, two-dimensional (e.g., 6-inch piece of paper) abstract representation of a much larger area, such as the Midwestern United States, including the roads running through that area. It might also include the exchange of numerical monetary information relating to the costs involved, which is also an abstract system. Finally, such a dialogue might include statements of opinion by either party as to whether potential sites along the journey would be interesting, expensive, etc. Typically, these ideas are exchanged between you and your friend rapidly and effortlessly through auditory-oral communication. Of course, the words used in the communication of thoughts and ideas are themselves abstract concepts—sound sequences that individuals in a shared culture have learned to associate with various objects, actions, descriptors, or modifiers.

Figure 1.1 provides a simplified overview of the various processes and systems involved in human communication. For clarity, only two individuals are depicted here: the talker and the listener or, more generally, the sender and the receiver of information. The sender has a thought or idea formulated in his or her mind and would like to convey this information to the mind of the receiver. This interactive network of the processes supporting such mind-to-mind communication is referred to here as the **communication chain.** This concept borrows heavily from the concept of the "speech chain," first introduced to the authors many years ago and still popular today (Denes & Pinson, 1963; 1993). The primary changes made to the original speech chain were to broaden it to include the exchange of visual information between the sender and the receiver. This visual information might be in the form of facial gestures that accompany speech production by the sender or the use of alternative modalities for communication, including manual forms of communication such as American Sign Language (ASL).

One important concept in Figure 1.1 is that there is a desire for the sender to send some information to the receiver; that is, to communicate some thoughts, ideas, or information. In typical auditory-oral communication, the exchange is initiated by the sender's brain organizing his or her thoughts to be

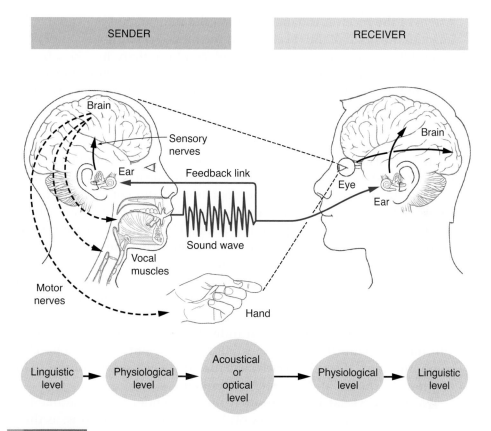

FIGURE 1.1 A schematic illustration of the communication chain between the "sender" and the "receiver." In typical auditory-oral communication, the sender is a talker and the receiver is a listener.

communicated, in the sender's acquired **language**, then directing the articulators of the speech mechanism (ranging from vocal cords at one end of the vocal tract to the lips at the other end) to produce a sequence of sounds associated with the words and grammar used in that language to communicate the intended message. (Further discussion of language processes can be found in Chapter 8.) In this case of typical auditory-oral communication, the primary link between the sender and receiver is the acoustic information generated by the sender. At this stage, hearing plays a critical role in the communication chain. The receiver's sensory system for hearing is used to encode the sound sequence spoken by the sender. This information from the hearing system is then sent via the nervous system to the brain of the receiver and decoded, assuming the receiver knows the language used by the sender. If the auditory system of the receiver is damaged, then the information may not be delivered intact to the brain of the receiver and the message may not be understood correctly. Of course, this is not the only place where there may be a break in the communication chain. For example, the sender may have impaired speech such that the acoustic stimulus sent to the receiver is degraded, which can hinder communication. Also, either the sender or the receiver may have higher-level cognitive or linguistic deficits that can degrade the message sent or the interpretation of the message received.

In this text, however, the primary breaks in the communication chain under consideration are those impacting the hearing of the sender or the receiver. In this regard, from the depiction of the communication chain in Figure 1.1, it is apparent that the receiver is not the only one who may be impacted negatively by impaired hearing. The sender's hearing system also encodes the spoken message as a way of monitoring the accuracy of the message and the sound sequence representing it. If the sender has impaired hearing, the way in which the sound sequence comprising the spoken message is produced may be impacted. Thus, hearing plays a critical role in deciphering the spoken message for the receiver and in the monitoring of the spoken message produced by the sender. An individual with impaired hearing may not only have difficulty hearing others, but may also contribute to a breakdown in communication through poorly articulated speech owing to the inability to monitor the quality of the speech generated.

Note that visual information from the sender is also available to the receiver, even in typical auditory-oral communication. That is, as the sender is moving the articulators to produce speech, visible cues for the identity of the sounds spoken are also provided to the receiver. The speech sounds /b/, /p/, and /m/, for example, are very visible and characterized by the rapid parting of the talker's lips. Similarly, the position of the lower teeth against the upper lip is a strong visual cue for the speech sounds /f/ and /v/. Not all speech sounds are as visible as these examples. Nonetheless, some individuals are very adept at using this additional visual information from the sender to help understand the spoken message so that they can understand the message. This may enable them to understand the message even when little acoustic energy from the spoken message is perceived by the receiver. Examples of conditions that require greater reliance on visible speech cues include high levels of background sound (noises, music, or other people talking), great distances between the sender and the receiver (perhaps even requiring devices such as binoculars to see the person speaking), or severely impaired hearing.

For some individuals, however, visual communication might be the primary means of communication between the sender and the receiver, rather than a supplement to the auditory information. This may again apply to persons with severe **hearing impairments** who use speechreading (also referred to as "lipreading") to perceive the message spoken by the sender. Some individuals with impaired hearing, especially many of those who developed the hearing impairment after spoken language had been acquired, can make good use of the visual cues in speech to enable very good "auditory-oral" communication. Speechreading ability is known to vary widely among individuals, however, and the factors that make one person a good speechreader and another seemingly similar person a poor speechreader are not well understood.

In other cases, communication between sender and receiver may make exclusive use of visual stimuli. An example of such a communication system in the United States is ASL. In this system, as illustrated schematically in Figure 1.1, sequences of finger, hand, and arm gestures comprise the primary link between the sender and the receiver. These hand gestures may be complemented by other visual or spatial cues, such as the spatial location of the hand gesture relative to the sender's location or accompanying facial gestures. As in typical auditory-oral communication, the communication sequence in manual communication is initiated in the mind of the sender. As noted in Figure 1.1, this, in turn, leads to signals from the brain of the sender to the motor nerves of the fingers, hands, arms, and face; this process then leads to a sequence of gestures conveying the message using the rules of the sender's language. These stimuli result in patterns seen by the receiver's visual system, which encodes the optical information and then sends it via the nervous system to the brain of the receiver. If the receiver knows the language used by the sender, this sequence of neural events is decoded by the receiver and the sent message is understood. Note here that mind-to-mind communication has taken place between the sender and the receiver while completely bypassing the auditory systems of both the sender and the receiver. Thus, manual communication in this fashion would be unaffected by hearing loss of any severity.

Of course, just as with typical auditory-oral communication, there are factors that might restrict the ability to communicate manually. It is critical, for instance, that the sender and receiver be able to see one another. Thus, manual communication with the sender in one room and the receiver in another is not possible without a direct visual link. Modern technology, however, such as the use of videophones or webcams, has made a visual link between the sender and receiver much less problematic when each is separated by great distances from the other (just as telephones have enabled auditory-oral communication over great distances).

Perhaps the most critical requirement for the successful use of manual communication, however, is that both the sender and receiver must be fluent in the specific manual language being used. In contemporary cultures worldwide, auditory-oral communication is used by the overwhelming majority of people. In these same cultures, the use of manual communication is primarily restricted to situations or circumstances in which auditory-oral communication is not readily accessible without the intervention of others. One such circumstance for which manual communication systems have been developed involves communication with and by profoundly hearing-impaired or Deaf individuals. Historically, the development of manual communication systems for Deaf individuals preceded the development of modern technologies, such as hearing aids and cochlear implants, designed to provide the Deaf with access to auditory-oral communication. Manual languages developed for and by Deaf individuals serve a limited segment of society and are not the "default" system in a specific society, societies dominated by hearing people. This is not to imply, however, that manual languages like ASL are impoverished or otherwise incapable of supporting the communication chain. To the contrary, ASL has been demonstrated to be a rich language capable of supporting the highest levels of abstract mind-to-mind communication. For such communication to take place, however, the sender and the receiver must be fluent in the language supporting mind-to-mind communication and, by sheer numbers alone, the overwhelming majority of individuals encountered in a given society are likely to be conversant in one of many spoken languages, rather than a manual language. This severely constrains the utility of manual languages, such as ASL, in broader society.

DEVELOPMENT OF THE COMMUNICATION CHAIN

Another key feature of the language system used for communication between the sender and the receiver is the manner in which language is usually acquired. Typically, language is acquired "naturally" through repeated exposures to the language early in life. Evidence suggests that the language-learning process itself is innate and early experience with language determines the specific language system that will be developed. Thus, most children born and raised in France learn French as their first language and, likewise, most of those born and raised in Italy learn Italian as their native language. The learning of a first language is usually a process in which the infant and toddler capitalizes on the pre-wired, innate, language-learning capabilities through repetitive exposures to language samples from members of the same language community, primarily the child's family, especially the mother. Within the context of the communication chain in Figure 1.1, the parent is the sender and knows the sequence of sound patterns associated with spoken words having various meanings and, through repetition of these same sound sequences in a variety of contexts, the child, as the receiver, begins to extract the code and develop an expanding vocabulary or lexicon, mapping sound patterns to various objects, actions, descriptors, or modifiers. Through frequent exposures, the child also learns the rules in the language that govern the order of such sound sequences in meaningful phrases or sentences (syntax). For communication to take place between the sender (parent) and the receiver (child), the receiver must develop the same code for deciphering the stream of sounds spoken by the sender. Otherwise, even with all other aspects of the communication chain functioning properly, communication between sender and receiver is not likely to take place.

Another aspect of this remarkable language-learning process is that it is a relatively rapid process. Table 1.1 lists some common language benchmarks for the development of typical auditory-oral communication. In general, the same developmental milestones have been observed for the development of ASL, at least for the case of Deaf children raised by Deaf parents. Clearly, language develops rapidly over the first 4 to 5 years of life when the young receiver is immersed in language produced by experienced senders (again, typically, the immediate family and primarily the mother).

Evidence supports the existence of a critical period for the development of a child's first language. As an upper bound for the limits to acquisition of typical language skills, it is generally believed that a child should know at least 50 to 100 words by the age of 5 to 7 years to have an opportunity to subsequently develop typical speech and language skills. Again, this is an upper age limit, and most children typically acquire this minimum proficiency *well before* the age of 5 years (typically, within the first year or two of life), as illustrated in

TABLE 1.1   Some General Milestones for Typical Speech and Language Development

Age (in years)	Milestone
1 year	Should have produced "first word"
2 years	Two-word phrases ("Daddy go")
	Expressive vocabulary of at least 40 words
	Receptive vocabulary of at least 50 words
4 years	Uses grammatically correct sentences
	Expressive vocabulary of at least 200 words
	Receptive vocabulary of at least 400 words
	95% of speech is adult-like and readily understood by others (including strangers)

Table 1.1. Again, they do so primarily through repetitive exposure to the language spoken by family members and members of the surrounding community. Once the child acquires the critical number of words in his or her lexicon or vocabulary, then the rules of grammar are developed to generate appropriate sequences of these words. For example, a young child acquiring spoken English will typically develop subject-verb or subject-verb-object word orders early in the use of sentences. Examples of such word orders include "Daddy go," "Baby cry," and "Puppy drink water." The key developmental trigger for the generation of meaningful strings of words in sentences appears to be the acquisition of a vocabulary of 50 to 100 words. If such a vocabulary size is not attained by an age of about 5 to 7 years, then future ability to generate meaningful sentences may be irreversibly impaired. In fact, there is some evidence from children raised in dire circumstances that indicates failure to acquire this minimum vocabulary size of 50 to 100 words by 11 to 12 years of age may result in a total inability to generate meaningful sentences as an adult (Vignette 1.1).

HEARING LOSS AND BREAKS IN THE COMMUNICATION CHAIN

For about 90% of the Deaf children born in the United States, both parents have normal hearing and their communication system is auditory-oral. This creates an immediate break in the communication chain between parents and the child. Figure 1.2 schematically illustrates this break in the communication chain when the child is the receiver and the parent is the sender of information. This is the most common direction of information exchange for the developing child and is discussed further below. Note here that the hearing-impaired child may not be able to monitor the quality of the vocal output being produced and that this may ultimately have a negative impact on the clarity of the child's speech. Deaf babies actually go through some of the same early stages of speech production (e.g., babbling) as typically developing auditory-oral babies. Without early intervention with hearing aids or cochlear implants, these early stages of speech production are not reinforced auditorily through subsequent imitation by the parent because the parent's mimicry "falls on deaf ears." As a result, the spontaneous vocal productions of profoundly hearing-impaired infants diminish in frequency and do not lead to the next stages of speech development observed in normal-hearing infants.

As noted, in the top panel of Figure 1.2, the receiver (the child) has a nonfunctional auditory pathway incapable of encoding the acoustic signals being

VIGNETTE 1.1   FURTHER DISCUSSION

FORBIDDEN EXPERIMENTS

How do scientists confirm the existence of possible critical periods for language development? One approach, the "forbidden experiment," would be to raise a child in complete isolation, without any language input or contact from others. One child could be isolated at 6 months of age, another child at 12 months of age, another at 18 months of age, and so on. The impact of isolation for various periods on speech and language development could then be studied. It is obvious why such an experiment is forbidden and could not be performed by scientists.

Unfortunately, from time to time, there have been naturally occurring "experiments" such as these where, through a terrible set of circumstances, children are raised in isolation for various periods of time. Perhaps two of the most well known such cases are Victor and Genie. Victor was the initial "wild child," apparently raised in isolation in the woods of France in the 1800s and not discovered by others until the age of about 12 years. Victor's story, and the attempts to restore speech and language, was popularized in the Francois Truffaut film, "The Wild Child *[L'Enfant Sauvage]*," released in 1970.

Coincidentally, at about the time this movie was being released, the case of Genie emerged in Los Angeles. Genie was discovered at the age of 13 years, having spent most of her life, since the age of about 18 months, raised by elderly parents who isolated her day and night in a small locked room, often tying her to a potty chair. The father, who was believed to be schizophrenic, apparently beat her whenever she vocalized, and she did not gain her freedom from these dire circumstances until her father's death. Genie's story was popularized in a variety of ways too, including a Public Broadcasting Service NOVA presentation in 1997 entitled, "Secret of the Wild Child." Although Genie could learn to communicate with a restricted vocabulary using isolated words or phrases, she never gained the ability to produce sentences and her language skills, despite extensive intervention, never approached "normal" levels.

Case studies of children, such as Victor and Genie, raised in dire circumstances and deprived of typical language input, have provided some of the evidence in support of the existence for a critical period for language acquisition. Because these "natural experiments" were not coordinated or conducted as empirical research, they offer only some general guidelines as to the nature and extent of the critical period.

generated by the senders (the parents), who are relying exclusively on an auditory-oral communication system. For communication to take place, and in this case, for language to develop from repetitive communication, there are two choices. The break in the communication chain at the auditory system of the receiver must be repaired (e.g., through medical treatment, a hearing aid, or a

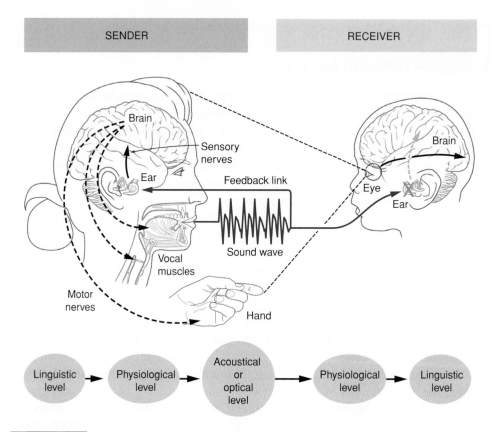

SENDER

RECEIVER

Brain

Sensory nerves

Ear

Feedback link

Sound wave

Vocal muscles

Motor nerves

Hand

Brain

Eye

Ear

Linguistic level → Physiological level → Acoustical or optical level → Physiological level → Linguistic level

FIGURE 1.2 Illustration of a break in the communication chain resulting from hearing loss. The break is illustrated in auditory periphery of the receiver (listener), who is a hearing-impaired child.

cochlear implant) or the sender must switch to a communication mode that does not rely on hearing (e.g., ASL). The parents, however, as the language models for their Deaf child, are not fluent in ASL or other forms of manual communication. Rather, in the United States, the parents are most likely to be fluent in spoken English or Spanish. The child, on the other hand, cannot hear the spoken English or Spanish messages being sent by the parents or other family members. As a result, there is a breakdown in communication and the child is not learning the language of the parents, or any language for that matter. Moreover, as noted previously, there is a critical period for the development of sufficient language proficiency to support adequate mind-to-mind communication. Thus, the clock is ticking for the resolution of this dilemma. Either the impaired auditory system of the child must be identified quickly and treated to enable the development of typical auditory-oral communication or the child must be immersed in ASL. The latter solution typically involves the parents learning ASL as a second language and frequently turning over their language-modeling roles to members of the Deaf community who are fluent in ASL.

Debates about the most effective resolution to this dilemma have raged for well over a century. Our perspective on this debate is as follows. First, regardless of the communication system to be used, the early identification of hearing impairment is critical. Without knowing the status of the child's hearing, it is not possible to intervene effectively, regardless of the path chosen. Second, for the overwhelming majority of profoundly hearing-impaired children, the 90% born to two normal-hearing parents, the default intervention should be restoration of hearing and reliance on auditory-oral communication rather than reliance on manual communication, although manual communication can be used as a supplement to auditory-oral communication as needed.

Our rationale for this stance is based on a number of practical circumstances rather than a clear superiority of auditory-oral language systems over manual language systems. For example, as indicated previously, the overwhelming majority of members in our society rely on auditory-oral forms of communication and, as noted in the discussion of the communication chain, effective communication requires knowledge of a common language by both the sender and the receiver. Thus, in most daily activities and encounters, a profoundly impaired person is more likely to encounter users of auditory-oral communication systems than manual communication systems. In addition, written languages for manual communication systems, such as ASL, do not exist at present. Consequently, the hearing-impaired person who learns ASL as the primary form of communication must learn a second language (e.g., English) for written communication and literacy. This is not the case, of course, when English is the choice for both written and spoken communication. In this case, there is greater redundancy between the acquisition of spoken and written language skills.

In addition, there is considerable evidence that communication, in either written or oral form, is less effective in a person's second language than in his or her first language. One way in which this has probably manifested itself has been in the long-standing observations of less than satisfactory reading and mathematics achievement scores for the Deaf population in the United States. Statistics from a national research institute at the only liberal arts college in the United States for the Deaf (Gallaudet Research Institute, 2005), for example, indicate that the average Deaf high-school graduate (Grade 12, or an age of 18 years) reads at a fourth-grade level on the Stanford Achievement Test

(SAT); actually, on a special version of the test adapted for use with individuals having impaired hearing (SAT-HI). Average mathematics scores on the SAT-HI are at the sixth-grade level for the same age group of Deaf individuals nationwide. Because the SAT-HI is administered in written English, at least part of the poor average performance may be due to a mismatch between the first language (ASL) of many of the test takers and the language of the test (written English). Nonetheless, to the extent that the test captures proficiency in reading and math when using written English, the written language in which the Deaf were educated and on which they will need to rely in daily life, it suggests that performance in written English is less than satisfactory. It is acknowledged that the presumption made here is that similar large-scale data from hearing-impaired children with early auditory-oral intervention and exposure to oral English at an early age will exceed these reading and mathematics competencies for the SAT-HI. Although there is encouraging research with profoundly hearing-impaired children who received cochlear implants at an early age to support this supposition, the data available from such children, especially for those who have now reached an age of 18 years, are too sparse to clearly substantiate this argument.

Finally, there are other beneficial byproducts of the child's reliance on auditory-oral communication that we consider to be beneficial to the person with impaired hearing. These include the ability to communicate with unseen senders and receivers (over the telephone, in other rooms, etc.), to simultaneously monitor multiple senders (talkers) in the same or different locations (while concurrently using the other modality, vision, to monitor yet another object or location), to hear a wide variety of audible warning and alerting sounds designed for safety and protection, and to appreciate other auditory stimuli involved in the communication of mood or other types of messages, such as instrumental and vocal music.

SUMMARY

The communication chain provides a general framework for the communication between a sender and a receiver and enables the ultimate human experience: mind-to-mind communication of feelings, thoughts, and ideas. For typical auditory-oral communication, the predominant modality for communication throughout the world, hearing plays a central role. Impaired hearing can have a negative impact on both the sender and the receiver in the communication chain. Breakdowns in communication may result. To minimize the impact of the hearing impairment on communication and its development, the hearing loss must first be detected as soon as possible after its onset (regardless of the individual's age). The best option for the overwhelming majority of children with impaired hearing is to restore communication by improving the individual's hearing as soon as possible so as to acquire or sustain typical auditory-oral communication abilities.

Given the foregoing, the subsequent chapters of this text assume the primacy of auditory-oral communication for the majority of hearing-impaired persons—the primary exception being Deaf children raised by Deaf parents and immersed in ASL and Deaf culture. As such, for the remainder of this book, it is assumed that the primary link between sender and receiver is the acoustic signal generated by the sender. The acoustic signal is the topic of Chapter 2. Subsequent chapters deal with the encoding of the acoustic stimulus within the auditory system by both the receiver and the sender, the impact of various hearing disorders on communication, methods to identify the presence of hearing problems, and options for treatment of hearing disorders to improve auditory-oral communication.

CHAPTER REVIEW QUESTIONS

1. The communication chain illustrated in Figure 1.1 shows two separate auditory systems, one for the sender or talker and one for the receiver or listener. Figure 1.2 illustrates a break in the communication chain arising from a disorder in the auditory system. How would communication be impacted if the auditory system of the receiver was damaged so that it was completely nonfunctional? What if it was only the auditory system of the sender that had been damaged or destroyed? What if the auditory systems of both the sender and receiver are completely damaged?

2. What differences in speech-language development might you expect between the following two cases, assuming no intervention has taken place to repair the breaks in their respective communication chains? Both individuals have a complete loss of hearing in both ears, but one person has been like this since birth and the other since an age of 4 years. Both individuals are 6 years old at the time of examination. What differences would you expect and why?

3. The authors have adopted the viewpoint in this text that for persons with profound hearing loss who are considered Deaf, auditory-oral communication is preferred over manual forms of communication, like ASL, in the overwhelming majority of cases. How do they support this position? Do you agree or disagree? Why?

REFERENCES AND SUGGESTED READINGS

Denes PB, Pinson EN. *The Speech Chain*. Edison, NJ: Bell Telephone Laboratories; 1963.

Denes PB, Pinson, EN. *The Speech Chain, 2nd edition*. New York: W.H. Freeman; 1993.

Gallaudet Research Institute. *Stanford Achievement Test, 10th edition. Form A, Norms Booklet for Deaf and Hard of Hearing Students*. Washington, DC: Gallaudet University, Gallaudet Research Institute; 2005.

CHAPTER 2

Sound: The Typical Link Between Sender and Receiver in the Communication Chain

CHAPTER OBJECTIVES

- To appreciate the importance of sound as the primary link between the talker and the listener in the communication chain;
- To understand how sound waves are represented in the time domain;
- To see that the same sound can also be described in the frequency domain to emphasize the specific frequencies that are included in sound; and
- To understand the representation of a sound wave's magnitude or amplitude in terms of a sound level expressed in decibels.

KEY TERMS AND DEFINITIONS

- **Sound wave:** A disturbance created in a medium, such as air, by a source of vibration.
- **Waveform:** A graphical description of the variation in a sound wave's amplitude as a function of time.
- **Spectrum:** A graphical description of the variation in a sound wave's amplitude and phase as a function of frequency.
- **Decibel:** The unit of measure used to describe the level or magnitude of a sound wave.

As noted in Chapter 1, the typical link between the sender and the receiver in the communication chain is via spoken speech—an acoustic signal. To better understand the impact of impaired hearing on communication, it is critical to obtain a basic understanding of sound, including speech sounds. This chapter begins with a discussion of selected characteristics of sound waves, which is followed by a section on the representation of sound in the time domain (its waveform) and the frequency domain (its spectrum). This chapter concludes with a brief description of the measurement of sound level in decibels (dB).

SOUND WAVES AND THEIR CHARACTERISTICS

The air we breathe is composed of millions of tiny air particles. The presence of these particles makes the production of a **sound wave** possible. This is made clear by the simple yet elegant experiment described in Vignette 2.1. The

VIGNETTE 2.1   EXPERIMENT

The equipment shown in the accompanying figure: can be used to demonstrate the importance of air particles, or some other medium, to the generalization of sound waves. An electric buzzer is placed within the jar. The jar is filled with air. When the buzzer is connected to the battery, one hears a buzzing sound originating from within the jar. Next, a vacuum is created within the jar by pumping out the air particles. When the buzzer is again connected to the battery, no sound is heard. One can see the metal components of the buzzer striking one another, yet no sound is heard. Sound waves cannot be produced without an appropriate medium, such as the air particles composing the atmosphere.

#4

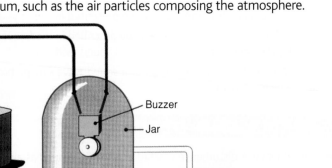

experiment demonstrates that air particles are needed for the production and transmission of sound in the atmosphere. There are approximately 400 billion air particles in every cubic inch of the atmosphere. The billions of particles composing the atmosphere are normally moving in a random fashion. These random continual movements of air particles make up what is known as *Brownian motion*. These random movements, however, can be ignored for the most part in our discussion of sound waves. It is sufficient to assume that each particle has an average initial or resting position.

When an object surrounded by air particles vibrates, the air particles adjacent to that object also vibrate. Thus, when a sufficient force is applied to the air particles by the moving object, the air particles will be moved or displaced in the direction of the applied force. Once the applied force is removed, a property of the air medium, known as its *elasticity*, returns the displaced particle to its resting state. The initial application of force sets up a chain of events in the surrounding air particles. This is depicted in Figure 2.1. The air particles

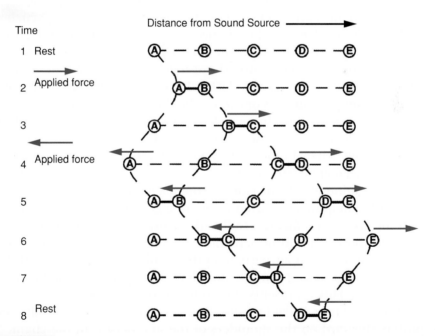

FIGURE 2.1   The movement of air particles (*A* through *E*) in response to an applied force at *t* = 2 and *t* = 4. The arrows indicate the direction of the applied force and the direction of particle displacement. Notice that each of the particles goes through a simple back-and-forth displacement. The wave propagates through the air, so that back-and-forth vibration of particle *A* eventually results in a similar back-and-forth vibration of particle *E*.

immediately adjacent to the moving object (labeled *A* in Fig. 2.1) are displaced in the direction of the applied force. They then collide with more remote air particles once they have been displaced. This collision displaces the more remote particles in the direction of the applied force. The elasticity of the air returns the air particles to their resting position. As the more remote particles are colliding with air particles still farther away from the vibrating object, force is applied to displace the object in the opposite direction. The void left by the former position of the object is filled by the adjacent air particles. This displaces the adjacent particle in the opposite direction. Note that the vibration of air particles passes on from one particle to another through this sequential series of collisions followed by a return to resting position. Thus, the displacement pattern produced by the object travels through the air particles via this chain of collisions.

Although we could measure this vibration in particles that are a considerable distance from the source of vibration, such as the particle labeled *E* in Figure 2.1, each particle in the chain of collisions has only moved a very small distance and then returned to its initial position. The air particles thus form the medium through which the vibration is carried. If the air particles adjacent to the vibrating object could actually be labeled, as is done in Figure 2.1, then it would be apparent that the vibration of air particles measured away from the vibrating object at point *E* would not involve the particles next to the object, labeled *A*. Rather, the particle labeled *A* remains adjacent to the object at all times and simply transmits or carries the displacement from resting position to the next air particle (*B*). In turn, *B* collides with *C*, *C* collides with *D*, *D* collides with *E*, and so on. A sound wave, therefore, is the movement or propagation of a disturbance (the vibration) through a medium, such as air, without permanent displacement of the particles.

Propagation of a disturbance through a medium can be demonstrated easily with the help of some friends. Six to eight persons should stand in a line, with the last person facing a wall and the others lined up behind that person. Each individual should be separated by slightly less than arm's length. Each person represents an air particle in the medium. Each individual should now place both hands firmly on the shoulders of the person immediately in front of him or her. This represents the coupling of one particle to another in the medium. Another individual should now apply some force to the medium by pushing forward on the shoulders of the first person in the chain. Note that the force applied at one end of the human chain produces a disturbance or wave that travels through the chain from one person to the next until the last person is pushed forward against the wall. The people in the chain remained in place, but the disturbance was propagated from one end of the medium to the other.

#3

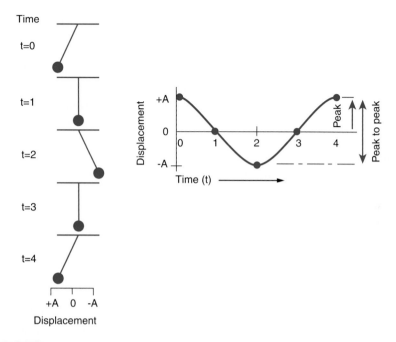

FIGURE 2.2 *Left,* Illustration of the movement of a pendulum at five instants in time, $t = 0$ through $t = 4$. *Right,* Notice that the simple back-and-forth vibration of the pendulum results in a sinusoidal waveform when displacement is plotted as a function of time.

Vibration consists of movement or displacement in more than one direction. Perhaps the most fundamental form of vibration is simple harmonic motion. Simple harmonic motion is illustrated by the pendulum in Figure 2.2. Note that the pendulum swings back and forth with the maximum displacement of A. The direction of displacement is indicated by the sign ($+$ or $-$) preceding the magnitude of displacement. Thus, $+A$ represents the maximum displacement of the pendulum to the left, 0 represents the resting position, and $-A$ represents the maximum displacement to the right. An object that vibrates in this manner in air will establish a similar back-and-forth vibration pattern in the adjacent air particles; the surrounding air particles will also undergo simple harmonic motion.

The five illustrations of the pendulum on the left side of Figure 2.2 show the position or the displacement of the pendulum at five different instants in time ($t = 0, 1, 2, 3,$ and 4). The plot in the right-hand portion of Figure 2.2 depicts the displacement as a function of time (t). Notice, for example, that at $t = 0$ the pendulum is displaced maximally to the left, resulting in a data point (dot) at +A for t = 0 on the graph in the right-hand portion of Figure 2.2. Similarly, at the next instant in time, t = 1, the pendulum returns to the resting position, or *0* displacement. This point is also plotted as a dot in the right-hand portion of Figure 2.2. The solid line connects the displacement values produced at each moment in time. If y represents the displacement, then this *solid line* can be represented mathematically by the equation y(t) = A sin (2π ft + φ). The details regarding this equation are not of concern here. The term t in this equation refers to various instants in time. Note that displacement and time are related to one another in this equation via the sine function. As a result, simple harmonic motion is often also referred to as sinusoidal motion or **waveform**; "sine wave" for short.

Another common physical system that is used to represent simple harmonic or sinusoidal motion is a simple mass attached to an elastic spring. Such a system can be oriented horizontally or vertically. An example of a horizontally oriented mass-spring system is shown in Figure 2.3. The top panel shows the mass-spring system at rest. Next, at t = 0, force is applied to displace the mass to the right and to stretch the spring. When this applied force is removed, the elasticity of the spring pulls the mass toward the original resting position (t = 1). The inertial force associated with the moving mass, however, propels the mass beyond the resting position until it is displaced to the left of the original resting position (t = 2). This results in a compression of the spring. When the elastic restoring force of the spring exceeds the inertial force associated with the moving object, the motion of the object is halted and begins in the opposite direction (t = 3). As the moving mass reaches the original resting position, inertial forces again propel it past the resting position until it has once again been fully displaced to the right (t = 4). Notice that the displacement of the mass and the stretching of the spring at t = 4 is identical to that seen at t = 0. One complete cycle of back-and-forth displacement has been completed. The sinusoidal equation used previously to describe the back-and-forth motion of the pendulum can also be applied to this simple mass-spring system.

The mass-spring system, however, is often easier to relate to air particles in a medium than a pendulum system. For instance, one can think of the mass in Figure 2.3 as an air particle, with the spring representing the particle's connection to adjacent air particles. In this sense, the movement of air particles described previously in Figure 2.1 can be thought of as a series of simple mass-spring systems like the one shown in Figure 2.3.

All vibration, including sinusoidal vibration, can be described in terms of its *amplitude* (A), *frequency* (f), and *phase* (φ). This is true for both the pendulum and the mass-spring system. The primary ways of expressing the amplitude or magnitude of displacement are as follows: (a) peak amplitude, (b) peak-to-peak

A cube (mass) attached to a spring which is attached to a wall at its other end. The mass is sliding back and forth across a surface (like a table top).

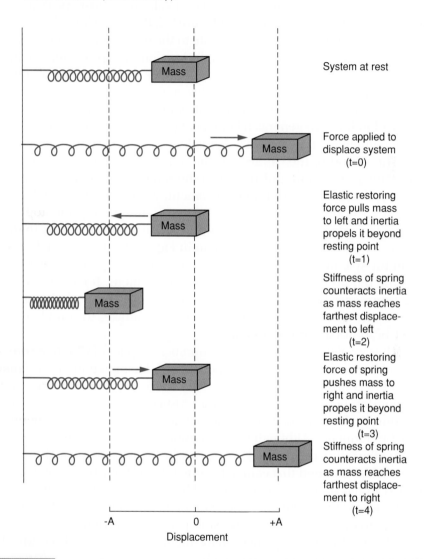

System at rest

Force applied to displace system
(t=0)

Elastic restoring force pulls mass to left and inertia propels it beyond resting point
(t=1)

Stiffness of spring counteracts inertia as mass reaches farthest displacement to left
(t=2)

Elastic restoring force of spring pushes mass to right and inertia propels it beyond resting point
(t=3)

Stiffness of spring counteracts inertia as mass reaches farthest displacement to right
(t=4)

-A   0   +A

Displacement

FIGURE 2.3   A simple mass-spring system in horizontal orientation is shown here to illustrate various stages of simple harmonic motion. The horizontal movement of the mass is depicted at five instants in time, $t = 0$ through $t = 4$. Notice that the simple back-and-forth vibration of this mass-spring system would result in a sinusoidal waveform of displacement as a function of time, just like the pendulum in Figure 2.2.

amplitude, and (c) root-mean-square (RMS) amplitude. RMS amplitude is an indicator of the average amplitude and facilitates comparisons of the amplitudes of different types of sound waves. The peak and peak-to-peak amplitudes are shown in the right-hand portion of Figure 2.2. Peak amplitude is the magnitude of the displacement from the resting state to the maximum amplitude. Peak-to-peak amplitude is the difference between the maximum displacement in one direction and the maximum displacement in the other direction. The amplitude of the sound can be considered to be roughly analogous to the perceptual attribute of loudness, although other characteristics of sound, including its duration, can impact loudness. In general, all else being equal between two sounds, a sound of higher amplitude is perceived as being louder than a sound of lower amplitude.

The period of the vibration is the time it takes for the pendulum to move from any given point and return to the same point. This describes one complete cycle of the pendulum's movement. Notice in Figure 2.2, for example, that at $t = 4$ the pendulum has returned to the same position it occupied at $t = 0$. The period in this case would be the difference in time between $t = 0$ and $t = 4$. For the mass-spring system in Figure 2.3, the time taken to progress from the system's state at $t = 0$ and to return to that state at $t = 4$ is the period or time required for one full cycle of displacement. If each interval in Figure 2.2 represented one-tenth of a second (0.1 s), the period would be 0.4 s. Hence, the period may be defined as the time it takes to complete one cycle of the vibration (seconds per cycle).

The frequency of vibration is the number of cycles of vibration completed in 1 second and is measured in cycles per second. Examination of the dimensions of period (seconds per cycle) and frequency (cycles per second) reflects a reciprocal relationship between these two characteristics of sinusoidal vibrations. This relationship can be expressed mathematically as $T = 1/f$ or $f = 1/T$, where $T =$ period and $f =$ frequency. Although the dimensions for frequency are cycles per second, a unit of measure defined as 1 cycle/s has been given the name hertz (Hz). Thus, a sinusoidal vibration that completed one full cycle of vibration in 0.04 s (i.e., $T = 0.04$ s) would have a frequency of 25 Hz ($f = 1/T = 1$ cycle/0.04 s). Although other factors contribute to the perceived pitch of sound, sound frequency can be thought to be roughly analogous to this perceptual attribute of sound. In general, sounds with higher frequencies have higher pitches and those with lower frequencies have lower perceived pitches.

Finally, the phase (φ) of the vibration can be used to describe the starting position of the pendulum or mass (starting phase) or the phase relationship between two vibrating pendulums or masses. Two sinusoidal vibrations could be created that were identical in amplitude and frequency, but different in phase, if one vibration started with the pendulum or mass in the extreme positive position (to the left) while the other began at the extreme negative

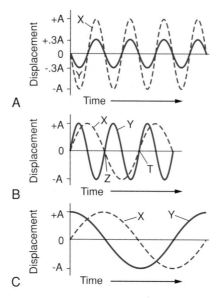

FIGURE 2.4 Sinusoidal waveforms differing only in amplitude (*A*), frequency (*B*), or starting phase (*C*).

displacement (to the right). In this case, the two pendulums or masses would be moving in opposite directions. This is called a 180-degree phase relationship. The two pendulums or masses could have the same amplitude of vibration (extent of back-and-forth movement) and move back and forth at the same rate (same frequency), yet still have different patterns of vibration if they failed to have identical starting phases.

Figure 2.4 contrasts the various features used to describe sinusoidal vibration. In Figure 2.4A, the two displacement patterns shown have identical frequencies and starting phases, but the amplitude of vibration is approximately three times larger for wave *X*. The peak amplitude of the vibration pattern labeled *X* is *A*, whereas that of pattern *Y* is 0.3*A*. In Figure 2.4B, on the other hand, amplitude and starting phase are equal, but the frequency of vibration for wave *Y* is twice as high as that for wave *X*. Notice, for example, that at the instant in time labeled *T* in Figure 2.4B, vibration pattern *X* has completed one full cycle of vibration, whereas pattern *Y* has completed two cycles at that same instant. Interestingly, although these two functions start in phase (both beginning at $t = 0$ with 0 displacement), their phase relationship is very complex at other instants in time. At the point labeled *Z* in Figure 2.4B, for example, the phase relationship is 180 degrees. Thus, at the moment in time labeled *Z*, both function *X* and function *Y* are at 0 displacement, but one is moving in a positive direction and the other in a negative direction. Figure 2.4C illustrates two functions of identical amplitude and frequency that differ only in their starting phase. To fully describe sinusoidal vibration, all three parameters—amplitude, frequency, and starting phase—must be specified.

In the initial discussion of the vibration of air particles, a situation was described in which force was applied to an object, which resulted in the object itself displacing adjacent air particles. When the force was removed, the object and the air particles returned to their resting positions. This was a case of forced vibration. Before describing the features of forced vibration in more detail, its counterpart, free vibration, deserves brief mention. In free vibration, as in the case of the pendulum or the mass-spring system described above, once the vibration is started by applying force, the vibration continues without additional force being required to sustain it. For free vibration, the form of the vibration is always sinusoidal, and the frequency of oscillation for a particular object is always the same. This frequency is known as the object's natural or resonant frequency (Vignette 2.2). The amplitude, moreover, can be no larger than the initial displacement. If there is no resistance to oppose the sinusoidal oscillation, then it will continue indefinitely. In the real world, however, this situation is never achieved. Friction opposes the vibration, which leads it to gradually decay in amplitude over time. To illustrate this, imagine that the mass depicted in the mass-spring system in Figure 2.3 is a smooth wooden cube that is sliding back and forth on a smooth glass surface. If the smooth glass surface is now replaced with a sheet of coarse sandpaper, then there will be greater friction created to oppose the back-and-forth movement of the block. The increased friction associated with the sandpaper surface will result in a quicker decay of the back-and-forth movement of the block in comparison with the original glass surface that offered much less resistance to the motion of the mass.

As illustrated in Vignette 2.2, objects with a specific mass and elasticity or stiffness will have a resonant frequency at which they prefer to vibrate. In speech communication, the vocal folds or vocal cords in the larynx represent a common example of this type of resonance in speech communication (Fig. 2.5). When air is forced through the vocal folds by the lungs, this causes them to vibrate at their natural frequency, which is determined by their mass and stiffness. As noted in Vignette 2.2, a system with higher mass, all else being equal between systems, will have a lower resonant frequency. The vocal folds of men, on average, have more mass than those of women, who, in turn, have vocal cords with more mass, on average, than those of children. As a result, the vocal cords typically have a lower resonant frequency in men than in women and in women than in children. It is this natural resonant frequency of the vocal folds, referred to as the fundamental frequency of the voice, that largely determines the pitch quality of voice. This is one of the primary reasons that

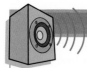

VIGNETTE 2.2   CONCEPTUAL DEMO

CONCEPTUAL ILLUSTRATIONS OF MASS, ELASTICITY, AND RESONANCE

You will be conducting a small experiment that requires the following materials: a yardstick (or meter stick), tape, four wooden blocks, and heavy-duty rubber bands.

Place two of the wooden blocks so that the ends of the blocks are flush with the end of the yardstick, one block on each side of the yardstick, and secure tightly with rubber bands. Hold or clamp about 6 inches of the other end of the yardstick firmly to the top of a table. Apply a downward force to the far end of the yardstick (the end with wooden blocks) to bend it down approximately one foot. (Don't push down too hard or the blocks may fly off of the yardstick when released.) Now release the far end of the yardstick, and count the number of complete up-and-down vibrations of the far end over a 10-second period. Repeat the measurements three times, and record the number of complete cycles of vibration during each 10-second period. This is experiment A.

Now add the other two wooden blocks to the end of the yardstick (two blocks on each side of the yardstick). Repeat the same procedure as above, and record the number of complete cycles three separate times. This is experiment B. If the number of complete cycles of vibration in each experiment is divided by 10 (for the 10-second measurement interval), the frequency (f) will be determined (in cycles per second). How has the system's natural or resonant frequency of vibration changed from experiment A to experiment B? By adding more blocks in experiment B, the mass of the system was increased. How was the system's natural or resonant frequency changed by increasing the mass of the system?

Now hold 18 inches of yardstick firmly against the table and repeat experiment B (4 wooden blocks). This is experiment C. This increases the stiffness of the system. How has the resonant frequency been affected by increasing the stiffness?

The resonant frequency of an object or a medium, such as an enclosed cavity of air, is determined largely by the mass and stiffness of the object or medium. Generally, stiffness opposes low-frequency vibrations, whereas mass opposes high-frequency vibrations. In the figure for this vignette, the *solid lines* show the opposition to vibration caused by mass and stiffness. The point at which these two functions cross indicates the resonant frequency of the system. The opposition to vibration caused by either mass or stiffness is the lowest at this frequency. The vibration amplitude is greatest at the resonant frequency because the opposition to vibration is at its minimum value. The *dashed line* shows the effects of increasing the mass of the system. Note that the resonant frequency (the crossover point of the *dashed line* and the *solid line* representing the stiffness) has been shifted to a lower frequency. The frequency of vibration in experiment B (more mass) should have been lower than that of experiment A. Similarly, if stiffness is increased, then the resonant frequency increases. The frequency in experiment C should have been greater than that in experiment B.

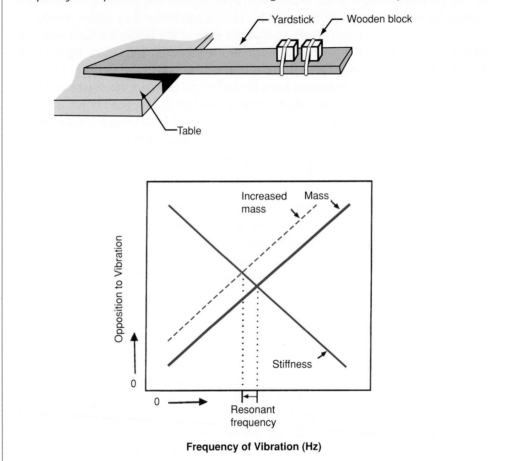

the pitch of men's voices sounds lower than that of women's voices, which, in turn, sound lower than that of children's voices.

This resonance involving mass and elasticity, however, is not the only type of resonance of interest in speech communication. Another type of resonance in acoustics that is of interest in speech communication is wavelength resonance. For our purposes, we will consider wavelength resonances as frequencies that are given preferential passage through air-filled tubes. Figure 2.6 illustrates a tube open at one end and closed at the other. If vibrations of various frequen-

Child

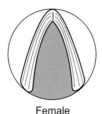

Female

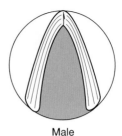

Male

FIGURE 2.5   The vocal folds of a typical child, adult woman, and adult man are illustrated here. Each is shown with the vocal folds open (blue air-filled space between them) and approximate the size of common U.S. coins (dime, nickel, and quarter, respectively). Assuming the stiffness or elasticity of each set of vocal folds is the same, then one of the primary changes in the vocal folds from children to women to men is an increase in mass. As noted in Vignette 2.2, such an increase in mass will result in a decrease in resonant frequency. Thus, on average, men have lower voice fundamental frequencies than women and women have lower fundamental frequencies than children. This largely, but not exclusively, determines the perceived pitch of the talker's voice.

cies and equal amplitudes are applied to the closed end of the tube, certain frequencies will pass through this tube better than others. The frequency that passes through this tube the best is the resonant frequency of that tube. The length of the tube is the primary determiner of the wavelength resonance for such tubes. In general, the shorter the length of the tube is, the higher the resonant frequency. A common example of this in music is the overall higher pitch produced by a piccolo compared to the overall lower pitch of the trombone. In addition, for a given musical instrument, such as the trombone, the length of the tube can be changed by the musician such that shorter tubes have higher resonant frequencies and give rise to higher pitches than longer tubes.

Figure 2.6 illustrates how the "tube closed at one end" applies to the generation of speech sounds. Basically, the air-filled spaces from the vocal cords (closed end) to the lips (open end) can be modeled as an air-filled tube closed at one end and open at the other. When the column of air in the tube is vibrated by the vocal cords at the closed end, certain frequencies are passed through this tube better than others. This column of air between the vocal cords and lips is typically referred to as the vocal tract; the average length in adult males is 17 cm. For a tube of this length, the resonant frequency is 500 Hz, with additional secondary resonances at 1500 and 2500 Hz. These resonant frequencies of the vocal tract are very close to those that have been recorded for men when producing the vowel /U/ (as in "hood"). This vowel is produced with close to a uniform diameter of the vocal tract from the vocal cords to the lips and is the

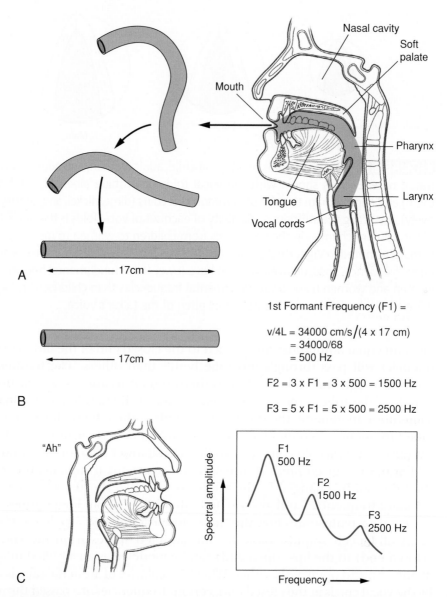

Nasal cavity

Soft palate

Mouth

Pharynx

Larynx

Tongue

Vocal cords

A ← 17cm →

B ← 17cm →

1st Formant Frequency (F1) =

v/4L = 34000 cm/s$/$(4 x 17 cm)
= 34000/68
= 500 Hz

F2 = 3 x F1 = 3 x 500 = 1500 Hz

F3 = 5 x F1 = 5 x 500 = 2500 Hz

"Ah"

Spectral amplitude

F1
500 Hz

F2
1500 Hz

F3
2500 Hz

Frequency →

C

FIGURE 2.6 Illustration of the modeling of the human vocal tract in an average male as a 17-cm tube open at one end (lips) and closed at the other (vocal cords). *A,* Relation of 17-cm tube to actual vocal tract. *B,* Calculation of quarter-wavelength resonant frequencies associated with the first three formant frequencies of the 17-cm vocal tract. *C,* Illustration of the acoustical measurement of the formant frequencies for the average male vocal tract when producing a vowel that results in a fairly uniform vocal tract (tube) diameter throughout. This is the speech situation that is closest to the 17-cm uniform diameter tube assumed when making the calculations and the measurements agree with the calculations.

English vowel that is closest to the "tube closed at one end" model. Other vowels may be generated by a given talker by changing the shape or length of the vocal tract in various ways such that the resonant frequencies are changed. Additional details are beyond the scope of this text. Note, however, that children will have shorter vocal tracts, on average, than women; women, in turn, will have shorter vocal tracts, on average, than men. Thus, for a given speech sound, such as the vowel /U/, this difference in vocal tract length will also contribute to the speech of children being higher in pitch than that of women and the speech of women being higher in pitch than that of men, on average.

In summary, there are two primary types of resonance that impact the speech signal forming the link between the talker and the listener. One resonance involves the mass and stiffness of the vocal cords and is the primary determiner of the pitch quality of the speaker's voice. The other resonance is a wavelength resonance involving the length and shape of the vocal tract. These resonances provide important clues as to the identity of the specific speech sound uttered by the talker and have a secondary influence on the overall pitch of the talker's voice. Together, both types of resonances shape the sound generated by the speaker and ultimately impact the sound perceived by the listener. We will return to these speech acoustics concepts shortly, but first we must continue our discussion of general acoustics.

Now that some general features of vibration, including resonance, have been reviewed, let us return to the discussion of sound generation and propagation. Consider the following situation. The force applied to an object surrounded by air particles is sinusoidal, resulting in a sinusoidal back-and-forth displacement of the surrounding air particles. The object displaces adjacent air particles in one direction, causing a temporary build-up or increase in density of the air particles. As the object returns to resting position because of its associated elastic restoring forces, the momentum associated with the mass of the object forces it past the resting state to its point of maximum displacement in the opposite direction. The immediately adjacent air particles attempt to fill the void left by the object, resulting in a less dense packing of air particles in this space. In doing so, the air particles surrounding the vibrating object undergo alternating periods of condensation and rarefaction. Therefore, the density of air particles is alternately increased and decreased relative to conditions at rest (no vibration). The increased concentration (density) of air particles results in an increase in air pressure according to a well-known law of physics, the ideal gas law. Thus, as the vibration propagates through the air medium, a volume of atmosphere goes through alternating periods of increased and decreased air particle density and, consequently, of high and low pressure. Waves of pressure fluctuations are created and travel through the medium.

Although the pressure variations associated with sound are small compared to normal atmospheric pressure for the air surrounding us, it is these small fluctuations in pressure that are important. The pressure fluctuations can be described using the same features discussed previously to describe changes in displacement over time. A sinusoidal driving force applied to an object vibrates the object and produces sinusoidal variations in pressure. These cyclic fluctuations in pressure can be described in terms of their amplitude, frequency, and phase. Pressure is the parameter most often used to describe sound waves because most measuring devices, such as microphones, respond to changes in sound pressure and the ear, beginning at the eardrum, responds to changes in pressure.

The unit of sound pressure is the *pascal* (Pa). Recall that the term *hertz*, rather than *cycles per second*, is used to describe the frequency of a sound. The use of the term *hertz* for frequency and the term *pascal* for sound pressure reflects the contemporary practice of naming units of measure after notable scientists (Vignette 2.3).

Unfortunately for the student, this practice often obscures the dimensions of the quantity. Pressure, however, is force per unit area and has frequently been described in units of either newtons (N) per meter squared or dynes (d) per centimeter squared. Vignette 2.4 explains why there are two different types of units for force, dynes versus newtons, as well as the use of various prefixes in the metric system to modify these or other physical units.

Although sound pressure is the preferred quantity for depicting the amplitude of a sound wave, another commonly used quantity is acoustic intensity. *Acoustic intensity* and *sound power* are used synonymously in this book. It is possible to derive the acoustic intensity corresponding to a given sound pressure. For our purposes, however, it will suffice that acoustic intensity (I) is directly proportional to sound pressure (p) squared: $I \equiv p^2$.

Let us suppose that a vibrating object completes two cycles of vibration when the appropriate driving force is applied. As the first condensation of air particles (or local high-pressure area) in the first cycle is created, it propagates through the medium and travels away from the source. During the second cycle of vibration, a new high-pressure area is created. By the time a second high-pressure area is completed, however, the first has traveled still farther from its point of origin. The *distance* between these two successive condensations or high-pressure areas is called the *wavelength* of the sound wave. (Recall that the *time* between successive condensations is the *period*.) If the frequency of vibration is high, the time interval between successive high pressure areas (the period) is short, and the separation between successive high-pressure areas is small. Given a short period, the first high-pressure area is unable to travel far from the source before the second high-pressure area arises. Thus, the wavelength—the separation in distance between successive high-pressure areas—is small. The wavelength (l), frequency (f), and speed of sound (c) are related in the following manner: $l = c/f$. Wavelength varies

VIGNETTE 2.3　HISTORICAL NOTE

UNITS OF SOUND NAMED AFTER FAMOUS SCIENTISTS

Hertz (*A*)

The unit of frequency, the hertz (Hz), is named in honor of Heinrich Rudolph Hertz, a German physicist born in 1857 in Hamburg. Much of his career was devoted to the theoretical study of electromagnetic waves. This theoretical work led eventually to the development of radio, an area in which frequency is very important. Hertz died in 1894.

Pascal (*B*)

The unit of sound pressure, the pascal (Pa), is named in honor of Blaise Pascal (1623–1662). Pascal was a French scientist and philosopher. He is well known for his contributions to both fields. As a scientist, he was both a physicist and a mathematician. In 1648, Pascal proved empirically that the mercury column in a barometer is affected by atmospheric pressure and not a vacuum, as was previously believed. Thus, his name is linked in history with research concerning the measurement of atmospheric pressure.

Newton (C)

The newton (N), the unit of force, is named in honor of the well-known English mathematician, physicist, and astronomer Sir Isaac Newton (1642–1727), who spent much of his career studying various aspects of force. Of his many discoveries and theories, perhaps the two best known are his investigations of gravitational forces and his three laws of motion.

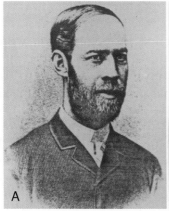
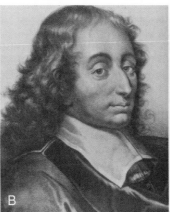
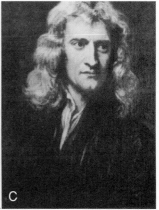

VIGNETTE 2.4   FURTHER DISCUSSION

REVIEW OF UNITS OF MEASURE AND METRIC PREFIXES

As mentioned in the text, one may encounter a variety of physical units for various physical quantities. For sound pressure, for example, units of N/m^2 or $dynes/cm^2$ may both be found in various sources. Although both of these units of pressure in this example are metric, one expresses area in meters and the other expresses area in centimeters. There are two basic measurement systems encountered in physics, the MKS system and the CGS system. The names for these two systems are derived from the units of measure within each system for the three primary physical quantities of length (meters in the MKS system and centimeters in the CGS system), mass (kilograms in the MKS system and grams in the CGS system), and time (seconds in both systems). The MKS system has been adopted as the standard international system for units of measure, so N/m^2 represents the preferred physical description of sound pressure. As noted previously, however, these physically meaningful units of force per unit area have been supplanted by units of Pascals (Pa).

In the metric system, the use of standard prefixes is commonplace. It is important, for a variety of auditory processes and measures, to have a good grasp on many typically used prefixes. The table below provides a listing of many such prefixes.

Prefixes for Fractions of a Unit			Prefixes for Multiple Units		
10^{-9}	nano (n)	0.000000001	10^9	giga (G)	1,000,000,000
10^{-6}	micro (μ)	0.000001	10^6	mega (M)	1,000,000
10^{-3}	milli (m)	0.001	10^3	kilo (k)	1,000
10^{-2}	centi (c)	0.01	10^2	hecto (h)	100
10^{-1}	deci (d)	0.1	10^1	deka (da)	10

inversely with frequency: the higher the frequency, the shorter the wavelength.

To clarify the concept of wavelength and its inverse relationship to frequency, consider once again the human chain that represented adjacent air particles. Suppose that, once a force was applied to the shoulders of the first person, it took 10 s for the disturbance (the push) to travel all the way to the end of the human chain. Let us also say that the chain had a length of 10 m. If a force was applied to the shoulders of the first person every 10 s, the frequency of vibration would be 0.1 Hz ($f = 1/T = 1/10$ s). Moreover, 10 s after the first push, the second push would be applied. Because we have stated that 10 s would be required for the disturbance to travel to the last person in the chain, when the second push is applied, the last person in the chain (10 m away) would also be pushing forward (on the wall). Thus, there would be a separation of 10 m between adjacent peaks of the disturbance or forward pushes. The wavelength (l) would be 10 m. If we double the frequency of the applied force to a value of 0.2 Hz, then the period is 5 s ($T = 1/f = 1/0.2 = 5$ s). Every 5 s, a new force will be applied to the shoulders of the first person in the chain. Because it takes 10 s for the disturbance to travel through the entire 10-m chain, after 5 s, the first disturbance will only be 5 m away as the second push is applied to the shoulders of the first person. Thus, the wavelength, or the separation between adjacent "pushes" in the medium, is 5 m. Notice that when the frequency of the applied force was doubled from 0.1 to 0.2 Hz, the wavelength

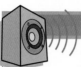

VIGNETTE 2.5 CONCEPTUAL DEMO

ILLUSTRATION OF THE PERIOD AND WAVELENGTH OF A WAVE

The figure below illustrates a giant wave pool, large enough to create waves for surfing. Waves in a wave pool are generated by displacing a wall at one end of the pool in a sinusoidal back and forth motion. The wave, once generated by the wall's displacement, travels through the water filling the wave pool. In the two top panels, the wall is moved back and forth at a higher frequency than in the two lower panels. In the left-hand panels, the surfers are sitting on their surf boards waiting to catch the crest of a wave. As they wait, they bob up and down in the water. When surfer A bobs up, we press a stopwatch and stop it when that same surfer bobs up again. This corresponds to the period of this wave. Which wave do you think has a shorter period? Since the wave in the top left panel has more waves or cycles per second (higher frequency) it has a shorter period, or fewer seconds per cycle (or wave).

In the right-hand panels, the three surfers each caught the crest of a successive wave and are riding it toward the far end of the wave pool. If we measured the distance between successive crests in the waves or, in this case, the distance between surfers riding those crests, we would find it to be a shorter distance in the top right panel than in the lower left panel. This separation of wave crests over distance corresponds to the wavelength for this wave. The higher the frequency, the closer the spacing of the wave crests over distance or the shorter the wavelength.

This analogy illustrates that the period can be considered to be the time separation of successive peaks of the sinusoidal waveform in seconds, whereas the wavelength is the length separation of successive peaks of the wave in meters. In both cases, the period and the wavelength are inversely related to the frequency of vibration. High frequencies yield short periods and short wavelengths, whereas low frequencies result in long periods and long wavelengths.

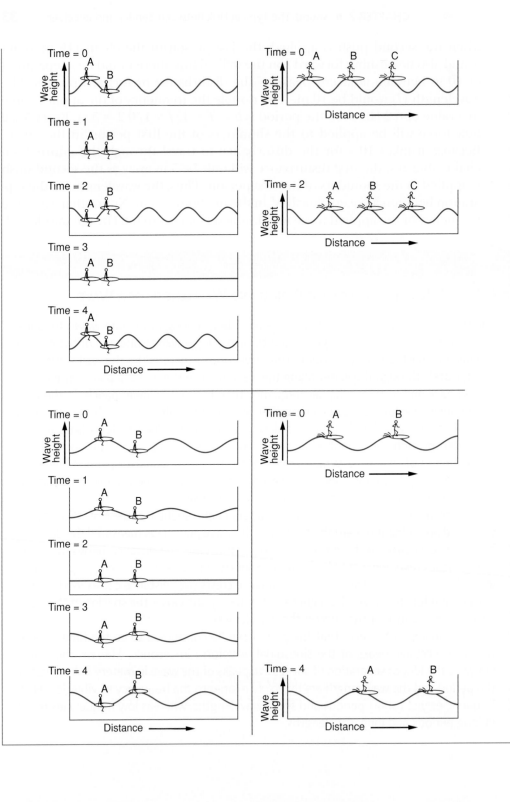

was halved from 10 m to 5 m. Frequency and wavelength are inversely related. Vignette 2.5 illustrates the concepts of a wave's period and wavelength.

Another feature of sound waves that is obvious to almost anyone with normal hearing is that the sound pressure decreases in amplitude as the distance it travels increases. It would be fruitless, for example, to attempt to hail a taxicab a half block away with a soft whisper even on a quiet street. Because the amplitude of sound decays with increasing distance, it would probably require high vocal effort to generate enough sound amplitude at the source to be audible to the cab driver a half block away. One would have to yell "Taxi!" rather than whisper it.

Under special measurement conditions, in which sound waves are not reflected from surrounding surfaces and the sound source is a special source, known as a *point source*, the decrease in sound pressure with distance is well defined. Specifically, as the distance from the sound source is doubled, the sound pressure is halved. Similarly, because of the relationship between sound pressure and acoustic intensity described previously ($I \equiv p^2$), the same doubling of distance would reduce the acoustic intensity to one-quarter [or $(1/2)^2$] the initial value. This well-defined dependence of sound pressure and sound intensity on distance is known as the *inverse square law*.

So far, we have considered some of the characteristics or features of a single sound wave originating from one source. Moreover, we have assumed that the sound wave was propagating through a special environment in which the wave is not reflected from surrounding surfaces. This type of environment, one without reflected sound waves, is known as a *free field*. A diffuse field is the complement of a free field. In a diffuse field, sound is reflected from many surfaces. The inverse square law that was just described holds true only for free-field conditions. In fact, in a diffuse field, sound pressure is distributed equally throughout the measurement area, so that no matter how far we go from the sound source or where we are in the measurement area, the sound pressure is the same. Typical classrooms are environments that lie somewhere between a free field and a diffuse field, probably closer to the latter in most cases. The term *sound field* is sometimes used to describe a region containing sound waves. Free fields and diffuse fields, then, are special classes of sound fields.

ANOTHER WAY TO LOOK AT SOUND WAVES: THE FREQUENCY DOMAIN

Many of the important features of a sound wave—such as its amplitude, frequency, and phase—can be summarized in either of two common formats. One

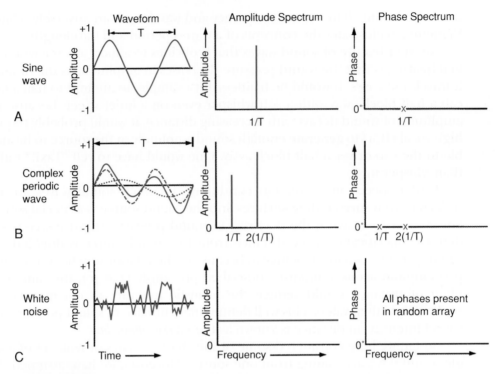

FIGURE 2.7 Illustration of the waveforms and corresponding amplitude and phase spectra for a continuous sine wave (*A*), a complex periodic wave (*B*), and white noise (*C*). All waveforms are assumed to be continuous, with only a brief snapshot of the waveform depicted here. In *B*, the *solid line* is complex waveform; *dashed* and *dotted* lines are the two sine waves making up the complex sound.

format, the **waveform**, describes the acoustic signal in terms of amplitude variations as a function of time. The sinusoidal waveform described previously for simple harmonic motion is an example of a waveform or time-domain representation of an acoustic signal. The term "time domain" simply reflects the fact that variations in time are shown along the x-axis in a plot of the waveform. For every waveform, there is an associated representation of that signal in the frequency domain, called the amplitude and phase **spectrum.** Here, "frequency domain" simply means that frequency is shown along the x-axis in this representation of sound. Figure 2.7A illustrates the amplitude and phase spectrum for a simple sinusoidal waveform. Note that the x axis of the spectrum is frequency, whereas the y axis is either amplitude or phase. The amplitude scale can be peak-to-peak amplitude, peak amplitude, or RMS amplitude, as noted previously. The phase spectrum, in this case, illustrates the starting phase of the acoustic signal. There can only be one possible waveform associated with the amplitude and phase spectrum shown in the right-hand side of Figure 2.7A. Similarly, there is only one set of amplitude and phase spectra associated with the waveform in the left-hand side of Figure 2.7A. Thus, both the time-domain and frequency-domain representation of the acoustic stimulus uniquely summarize its features. Furthermore, knowing one, we can derive the other. For every waveform, there is only one amplitude spectrum and phase spectrum associated with it. For every amplitude and phase spectrum, there is only one possible waveform. Vignette 2.6 uses an analogy to reinforce the notion that the waveform and the spectrum are just two different ways of looking at any given sound. On some occasions, it is the frequency content of a sound that we wish to focus on and the frequency domain provides an immediate indication of the frequencies comprising a sound, as well as their relative amplitudes and phases. On other occasions, it is the variations in amplitude over time that are of primary interest and examining sound in the time domain is most appropriate.

4 tones

Simple sinusoidal sounds are more the exception than the rule in everyday encounters with sound. Although sine waves have all of their amplitude at one and only one frequency, most everyday sounds have amplitude at more than one frequency. Fortunately, well over a century ago, a mathematician named Fourier determined that all complex periodic sounds consisted of a sum of simple sinusoids. A periodic sound is one in which the waveform repeats itself every T seconds. In the left-hand portion of Figure 2.7B, a complex periodic waveform is illustrated by the solid line. The dashed and dotted waveforms illustrate the two sinusoidal signals that, when added together, yield the complex sound. The spectrum of the complex sound can be represented by the sum of the spectra of both sinusoidal components, as illustrated in the right-hand portion of Figure 2.7B. Complex periodic sounds, such as that shown in Figure 2.7B, have a special type of amplitude spectrum known as line spectra. The amplitude spectrum consists of a series of discrete vertical lines located at various frequencies and having specified amplitudes. Each line represents a separate sinusoidal component of the complex sound. The component having the lowest frequency is called the *fundamental frequency*. The fundamental frequency corresponds to $1/T$, where T is the period of the complex sound. Additional components, located at frequencies corresponding to integer multiples of the fundamental frequency, are referred to as *harmonics* of the fundamental. If the fundamental frequency is 200 Hz, for example, then the second and third harmonics of 200 Hz are 400 Hz (2 × 200 Hz) and 600 Hz (3 × 200 Hz), respectively. The first harmonic corresponds to the fundamental frequency. Additionally, the term *octave* means a doubling of frequency. Continuing the same example, 400 Hz would be 1 octave above the fundamental frequency (200 Hz), whereas 800 Hz would be 2 octaves (another doubling) above the fundamental frequency.

4 tones
added

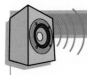

VIGNETTE 2.6   CONCEPTUAL DEMO

TIME-DOMAIN AND FREQUENCY-DOMAIN REPRESENTATIONS OF SOUND: AN ANALOGY USING MAPS

As noted in the text, sound can be represented completely and equivalently in two different fashions: the time domain, or waveform, and the frequency domain, or spectrum. It is important to realize that these displays of sound just offer two different "pictures" of the same sound. By analogy, consider the piece of the Earth known as the state of Indiana in the United States. As shown in this figure, there are many ways one could display the features of this piece of property. The map on the left is a road map for Indiana. The map in the middle depicts the average annual rainfall in the state and the one on the right illustrates the relative elevation of various portions of the land within the state. Each map serves a specific purpose and function, but all three represent information about *the same* piece of the Earth, Indiana. If the reader wanted to know the best route to take from Indianapolis, Indiana to Fort Wayne, Indiana, for example, the road map would be the map of choice. The road map, however, conveys no information about annual rainfall or topography. If this information is of interest to the reader, then the other maps would need to be consulted. This is similar to the choices available for the analysis and display of sound. If the moment to moment variations in the amplitude of a sound are of interest, the waveform is the most appropriate representation. Likewise, if the frequency content of the sound is of interest, then the amplitude and phase spectra would be the most appropriate displays. In either case, the sound would be the same, but the "picture" of that sound could be displayed in either the time-domain or frequency-domain format.

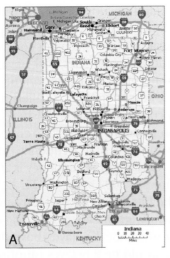
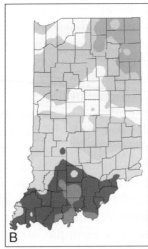
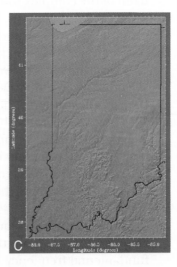

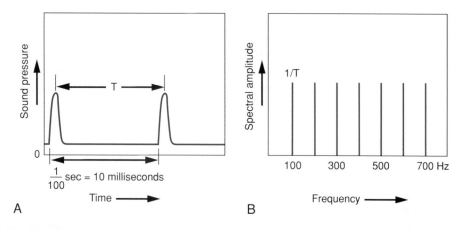

FIGURE 2.8   The waveform (*A*) and amplitude spectrum (*B*) of a series of glottal pulses measured (hypothetically) just above the vocal cords during voicing. Every time the vocal cords burst open from the air pressure generated by the lungs, the sound pressure increases rapidly and then decreases rapidly when the vocal cords close, as illustrated by the waveform in (*A*). The pulse repeats itself every 0.01 second. The corresponding amplitude spectrum (*B*) shows a series of vertical lines, beginning with the fundamental frequency [$1/T = 1/(0.01$ s/cycle$) = 100$ Hz] and including all harmonics (integer multiples) of the fundamental frequency (200, 300, 400 Hz . . .) at equal amplitude. It is this complex periodic sound generated by the vocal cords for voiced speech sounds, such as vowels, that is subsequently shaped by the resonances of the vocal tract. The fundamental frequency, in this case 100 Hz, is the primary determiner of the pitch of the talker's voice.

Figure 2.8 shows the waveform (left) and spectrum (right) for a hypothetical sound wave recorded by a microphone positioned just above the vocal cords. Notice that the waveform is essentially periodic (referred to as *quasi-periodic* because there are typically minor cycle-to-cycle variations), but more complex than a simple sine wave. The period of this waveform (*T*) is 10 ms or 0.01 s. This informs us that the lowest frequency in this sound, the fundamental frequency, is 100 Hz (1/0.01 s) and this is most likely the voice of a man. However, what other frequencies are in the waveform in the upper portion of Figure 2.8? It is not easy to tell by looking at it. The corresponding representation of this sound in the frequency domain, however (shown in the right-hand panel of Fig. 2.8), immediately reveals the frequencies that are in this sound and their relative amplitudes. Note that each frequency in this periodic sound is represented by a vertical line with the horizontal location on the x-axis indicating its frequency and the vertical height of each line represents the amplitude at that frequency.

For simplicity, we have omitted the display of phase information at each frequency (i.e., the phase spectrum), but it should be remembered that without this information it would not be possible to go back and forth between the time-domain and frequency-domain versions of the sound. Also note that individual lines are positioned at the harmonics of the fundamental frequency. This particular sound has energy at all of the harmonics above the fundamental frequency (100, 200, 300, 400 Hz...), but this is not always the case for complex waveforms. The key point illustrated in Figure 2.8 is that, although the waveform (left panel) and amplitude spectrum (right panel) provide equivalent depictions of sound, if the frequency content is the sound characteristic of interest, the amplitude spectrum provides an immediate illustration of this characteristic.

Figure 2.9 shows some additional waveforms and amplitude spectra for periodic vowel sounds. The left-hand panels depict various speech waveforms for individual vowels and the right-hand panels show the corresponding amplitude spectra for a brief sample of the vowel sound at one instant in time. In the top two pairs of panels (*A* and *B*), notice that the period (*T*) of the waveform is longer in the top panel and shorter in the middle panel. As a result, the talker's voice is considerably higher in pitch for the middle panel than the top panel. This is also illustrated by the vertical lines in the corresponding amplitude spectra on the right. Notice that the first (lowest frequency) vertical component is lower in the top panel than in the middle panel. The fundamental frequency is 100 Hz for the top panel and 300 Hz for the middle panel. This also results in the other vertical lines in the amplitude spectrum at higher harmonics being more widely spaced in the middle panel than in the top panel. Notice, however, that the resonant peaks or the formant frequencies (F1 to F3) for this speech sound are identical. These formant frequencies correspond to those in the vowel /a/. Thus, based on the pattern of formant peaks in the amplitude spectra on the right, it is apparent that the same speech sound, /a/, is being spoken by two different voices or talkers, most likely a male adult (fundamental frequency = 100 Hz) and a young child (fundamental frequency = 300 Hz).

The bottom pair of panels in Figure 2.9 depicts the waveform and corresponding amplitude spectrum for another sample of speech. How do these compare to the pairs in the middle and top panels of Figure 2.9? Regarding the waveforms on the left, the period (*T*) is the same as that in the top panel. Therefore, the fundamental frequency and pitch of the voice are the same in the top and bottom panels. This is also revealed in the narrow spacing of the vertical lines in the amplitude spectrum on the right. Note, however, that the pattern of formant frequencies and amplitudes (F1 to F3) differs between the top and bottom amplitude spectra. The bottom panel represents the vowel /U/ (as in "hood") spoken by the same talker producing the vowel /a/ ("ah")

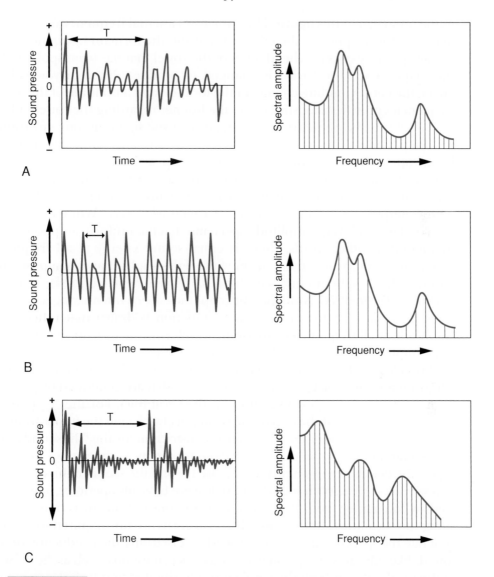

FIGURE 2.9 Illustrations of the differences between fundamental frequency and formant frequency. The left-hand panels show the waveforms for various speech sounds and the right-hand panels illustrate the corresponding amplitude spectra at one moment in time. Adapted from Denes & Pinson (1993).

in the top panel of this figure. Thus, the fundamental frequency $(1/T)$ is a primary cue for the pitch of the talker's voice and the formant frequencies (F1 to F3) are primary cues for the identity of the vowel that has been spoken. When the shape of the vocal tract is changed to produce different vowels by the talker, the corresponding change in the location and amplitude of the formant frequencies provides acoustic cues to the listener regarding the vowel's identity.

Vowel sounds are periodic, but many acoustic signals in our environment are not periodic. Noise is probably the most common example. Noise is said to be an aperiodic signal because it fails to repeat itself at regular intervals. Rather, the waveform for noise shows amplitude varying randomly over time. This is illustrated in the left-hand portion of Figure 2.7C. The case shown here is an example of a special type of noise called *white noise*. White noise is characterized by an average amplitude spectrum that has uniform amplitude across frequency; in other words, there is equal sound energy at all frequencies. (White noise derives its name from white light—light that is composed of all wavelengths of light at equal amplitudes.) This is depicted in the right-hand portion of Figure 2.7C. Note that the amplitude spectrum no longer consists of a series of lines. Rather, a continuous function is drawn that reflects equal amplitude at all frequencies. Aperiodic waveforms, such as noise, have continuous amplitude spectra, not discrete line spectra.

Speech sounds are also often comprised of noises. For example, the "f" and "sh" sounds in the word *fish* are basically noises that are generated by passing air from the lungs through constrictions in the vocal tract. For the "f" sound, the constriction is made at the end of the vocal tract by placing the upper front teeth in contact with the lower lip, whereas the constriction for the "sh" sound is made by arching the tongue so that it is in close proximity to the roof of the mouth. Again, the details of speech production are beyond the scope of this text. Suffice it to say that some speech sounds in English are basically aperiodic noises generated by forcing air from the lungs through constrictions in various locations along the vocal tract. In this case, the vocal cords are not required to vibrate to generate the speech sound, as was true when discussing the production of vowel sounds like "ah." It is also possible for some speech sounds, such as the "v" sound in the word *vat*, that both the vocal cords are vibrated and turbulence is generated as the vibrated air passes through a constriction in the vocal tract.

The acoustic speech signal is a very complex stimulus. The most complete picture of the speech signal is provided by looking at amplitude variations in both the frequency domain and time domain simultaneously. When this form of acoustic analysis is applied to speech stimuli, it is referred to as a *speech spectrogram*. Figure 2.10 (top) provides an illustration of a speech spectrogram for the phrase "the communication chain." For speech spectrograms, the y-axis is sound frequency, with lower frequencies at the bottom and higher frequencies

White Noise

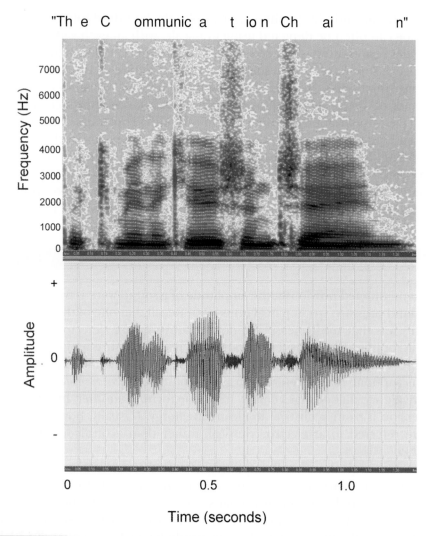

FIGURE 2.10 A speech spectrogram (top) and wakeform (bottom) for the utterance, "the communication chain," illustrating the complex acoustic code sent from the talker to the listener. The spacing of the phase at the top corresponds to the approximate locations of those speech sounds in the spectrogram and waveform.

at the top, and the x-axis is time. To represent the important third dimension in this analysis of speech sounds, amplitude, gradients of color or of grey are used to reflect the amplitude at a particular frequency and moment in time. Figure 2.10 shows a grayscale version of the speech spectrogram with shades of gray representing variations in amplitude. On this scale, black is the highest amplitude and white is the lowest amplitude. Hundred-fold variations in amplitude can often be depicted using grayscale, with an even wider range of amplitudes represented when color is used. Through detailed acoustical analyses of speech-sound patterns, such as those in Figure 2.10, and corresponding experiments on the perception of these sounds, researchers have identified many of the cues needed to recognize speech sounds produced by the speaker. In fact, under good listening conditions and a constrained set of communication contexts, computer algorithms have been developed that will accurately identify 90% of the speech spoken clearly into a microphone. Interesting research is also being conducted on the use of complex acoustic codes for communication among animals; some of the tools used to analyze human speech, such as the spectrogram, have also been applied in this area (Vignette 2.7).

SOUND MEASUREMENT

As mentioned previously, the amplitude of a sound wave is typically expressed as sound pressure (p) in pascal units (Pa). Recall that one of the major reasons for this was that most measuring devices are pressure detectors. Devices such as microphones are sensitive to variations in air pressure and convert these pressure variations to variations in electrical voltage. In more general terms, the microphone can be referred to as an *acousticoelectrical transducer*. A transducer is any device that changes energy from one form to another. In this case, the conversion is from acoustical to electrical energy. (Usually, however, microphones are referred to as electroacoustical, rather than acousticoelectrical, transducers.)

Although the overall amplitude of sound waves is best expressed in terms of RMS pressure, the use of the actual physical units to describe the level of sound is cumbersome. In humans, the ratio of the highest tolerable sound pressure to the sound pressure that can just be heard exceeds 10,000,000:1. Moreover, the units dictate that one would be dealing frequently with numbers much smaller than 1. The lowest sound pressure that can just be heard by an average young adult with normal hearing, for instance, is approximately 0.00002 Pa (2×10^{-5} Pa) or 20 μPa (micropascals).

Rather than deal with this cumbersome system based on the physical units of pressure, scientists devised a scale known as the **decibel** scale. The decibel scale quantifies the sound level by taking the logarithm (base 10) of the ratio of two sound pressures and multiplying it by 20. The following formula is used to calculate the sound level in decibels (dB) from the ratio of two sound pressures (p_1 and p_2): $20 \log_{10} (p_1/p_2)$. Let's use the range of sound pressures from maximum tolerable (200,000,000 μPa) to just audible (20 μPa) to see how this range would be represented in decibels. To do this, we begin by substituting

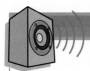

VIGNETTE 2.7 CONCEPTUAL DEMO

ACOUSTIC CODES FOR COMMUNICATION

Humans use complex acoustic information or codes to communicate. As noted in the text, these codes can be analyzed in terms of the sound's waveform, spectrum, or a combination of both—the spectrogram. Are humans the only animals to use acoustic information to communicate? No. Many species use sound to communicate warnings for perceived threats such as approaching predators, intentions such as aggression or submission, or location such as when locating a suitable mate for reproduction.

Some animals appear to make use of even more complex acoustic codes and for more elaborate forms of communication. The acoustic productions of the bottlenose dolphin, for example, have been studied extensively. One interesting sound generated by the bottlenose dolphin is referred to as a "signature whistle." This sound is believed to be unique to each dolphin's social group and, perhaps, to each individual dolphin; similar to the identifiers used by humans in communication ("I'm Larry Humes from Bloomington, Indiana.")

The figure below shows examples of three signature whistles recorded from three bottlenose dolphins. The top panel of each pair shows the waveform for the signature whistle whereas the bottom panel of each pair displays the corresponding sound spectrogram. Clearly, each waveform and spectrogram reveals a complex acoustic code and one that is unique for each of the three animals. By manipulating these signature whistles with a computer, researchers were able to basically change the voice (fundamental frequency) while leaving the shape of the sound spectrogram unchanged. This is roughly equivalent to having different talkers speak the same vowel sounds (Fig. 2.6) or words. Dolphins were able to recognize the signature whistles produced by different "voices" as well as the originals. Thus, bottlenose dolphins appear to be able to use complex acoustic signals as labels or identifiers of specific individuals, whether the identifier is produced by that animal or another animal; just as humans can understand the sound sequence that corresponds to "Larry Humes from Bloomington, Indiana," whether spoken by Larry Humes or someone else referring to him.

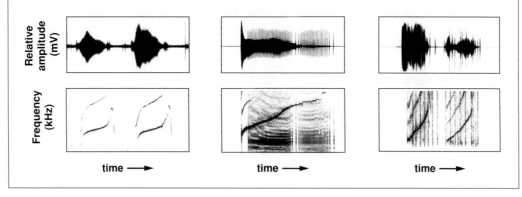

200,000,000/20 for p_1/p_2, which reduces to a ratio of 10,000,000/1. The $\log_{10}$ of 10,000,000 (or 10^7) is 7. When the number 7 is multiplied by 20, the result is 140 dB. This represents the maximum tolerable sound level. Now, for the just audible sound pressure of 20 μPa, the ratio of p_1/p_2 is 20/20, or 1. The log of 1 is 0, and 20 × 0 is 0. Thus, the just-audible sound pressure is represented by a sound level of 0 dB. We have taken a scale represented by a range of physical sound pressures of 200,000,000:20 and compressed it to a much more manageable range of 140 to 0 dB. The greatest sound pressure that can be tolerated is 140 dB larger than the softest sound pressure that can be heard. Note that this statement does not indicate what either of those sound pressures is in pascal units, which is because a ratio of two sound pressures has been used in the calculation of decibels and ratios are dimensionless quantities (e.g., 0.2 Pa/ 0.2 Pa = 1; *not* 1 Pa). Thus, we are calculating the decibel increase of one sound relative to another. Sometimes all we are interested in is a relative change in sound pressure. Recall from the discussion of the inverse square law, for example, that as the distance was doubled from the sound source, the sound pressure was decreased to half its original value. The corresponding change in decibels associated with this halving of sound pressure can be calculated by using a ratio of 0.5/1. The $\log_{10}$ of 0.5 is -0.301, which, when multiplied by 20, yields a change in sound pressure of approximately -6 dB. We can restate the inverse square law by indicating that, as the distance from the sound source is doubled, the sound pressure level decreases by 6 dB. Again, this does not indicate what the values are for the two sound pressures involved in this change. The sound pressure may begin at 10 Pa and be halved to 5 Pa or may start at 10,000 Pa and decrease to 5,000 Pa. Either of these cases corresponds to a halving of the initial sound pressure, which corresponds to a 6-dB decrease in sound level.

Often, an indication of the sound pressure level, which provides an absolute rather than a relative indication of the sound level, is needed. To accomplish this, all sound pressures relative to the same reference sound pressure must be evaluated. Thus, the denominator of the decibel equation becomes a fixed value called the *reference sound pressure*. The reference sound pressure for a scale known as the sound pressure level (SPL) scale is 2×10^{-5} Pa, or 20 μPa. As noted above, this corresponds to the softest sound pressure that can be heard by humans under ideal conditions. Calculation of the SPL for a specific sound pressure (p_1) can be accomplished by solving the following equation: SPL in dB $= 20 \log [p_1/(2 \times 10^{-5}$ Pa$)]$. Perhaps the simplest case to consider is the lowest sound pressure that can just be heard: 2×10^{-5} Pa. If $p_1 = 2 \times 10^{-5}$ Pa, then the ratio formed by the two sound pressures is $(2 \times 10^{-5}$ Pa$)/(2 \times 10^{-5}$ Pa$)$, or 1. The log of 1 is 0, which, when multiplied by 20, yields a sound level of 0 dB SPL. Consequently, 0 dB SPL does not mean absence of sound. Rather, it simply corresponds to a sound with a sound pressure of 2×10^{-5} Pa.

Sound pressures lower than this value will yield negative dB SPL values, whereas sound pressures greater than this yield positive values.

Let us consider another example: A sound pressure of 1 Pa corresponds to how many decibels SPL? This can be restated by asking the reader to solve the following equation: SPL in dB = 20 log [1.0 Pa/(2 × 10^{-5} Pa)]. We begin by first reducing $1.0/(2 × 10^{-5})$ to $5 × 10^4$. The log of $5 × 10^4$ is approximately 4.7, which, when multiplied by 20, yields a sound pressure level of 94 dB. Thus, a sound pressure of 1 Pa yields a sound pressure level of 94 dB SPL. This sound level is within the range of typical noise levels encountered in many factories and would be perceived to be quite loud.

Fortunately, laborious calculations are not required every time measurements of sound pressure level are required. Rather, simple devices have been constructed to measure the level of various acoustic signals in decibels SPL. These devices, known as sound level meters, use a microphone to change the sound pressure variations to electrical voltage variations. The RMS amplitude of these voltage variations is then determined within the electronic circuitry of the meter, and an indicator (e.g., needle, pointer, or digital display) responds accordingly. In the case of 1 Pa RMS sound pressure input to the microphone, for example, the meter would either point to or display a value of 94 dB SPL (Vignette 2.8).

SUMMARY

The fundamentals of acoustics were reviewed in this chapter. Understanding the basics of sound is critical because sound waves form the primary link between the sender and receiver in the communication chain. We began the review of basic acoustics with simple harmonic motion or sinusoidal vibration, the simplest of all periodic sounds. The effects of varying the amplitude, frequency, and starting phase of the sinusoidal waveform were examined. The relation between the representations of sound in the time domain, the waveform, and sound in the frequency domain, the amplitude and phase spectra, were then reviewed. Resonance was also discussed. Special emphasis was placed on the complex acoustic code representing human speech. Finally, the measurement of sound levels in decibels was reviewed.

VIGNETTE 2.8   FURTHER DISCUSSION

DECIBEL VALUES OF COMMON SOUNDS

Sound Level	Common Sound at this dB level	
0 dB SPL	softest sound level heard by average human listener	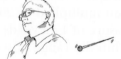
20 dB SPL	leaves rustling in a breeze	
40 dB SPL	whispered speech measured 1m away	
60 dB SPL	average, conversational speech measured 1m away	
80 dB SPL	loud, shouting voice measured 1m away	
100 dB SPL	city subway, nearby thunder	
120 dB SPL	typical level at a rock concert for audience	
140 dB SPL	jet engine at takeoff	

CHAPTER REVIEW QUESTIONS

1. Draw the waveform and amplitude spectrum for a sine wave or pure tone that has a peak amplitude of 10, a frequency of 1,000 Hz, and a starting phase of 0 degrees. Label all axes. What is the period for this sine wave?

2. Draw the waveform and amplitude spectrum for a sine wave that has half the amplitude and twice the frequency of the sine wave in Question 1 (starting phase remains at 0 degrees). Label all axes. What is the period of this sine wave?

3. Draw the waveform and amplitude spectrum for a sine wave that has half the amplitude and twice the frequency of the sine wave in Question 2 (starting phase remains at 0 degrees). Label all axes. What is the period of this sine wave?

4. Compare your answers to Questions 1 to 3. What happened to the period of the sine wave as the frequency was doubled (increased by 1 octave)? Why?

5. Assume that the amplitude axis for Questions 1 to 3 is in units of sound pressure (Pascals). How would the sound level in dB SPL change as one progressed from Question 1 to Question 2 and from Question 2 to Question 3?

REFERENCES AND SUGGESTED READINGS

Beranek LL. *Acoustics.* New York: McGraw-Hill; 1954.

Berlin CI. *Programmed Instruction on the Decibel.* New Orleans: Kresge Hearing Research Laboratory of the South, Louisiana State University School of Medicine; 1970.

Cudahy E. *Introduction to Instrumentation in Speech and Hearing.* Baltimore: Williams & Wilkins; 1988.

Denes PB, Pinson EN. *The Speech Chain.* New York: WH Freeman; 1993.

Durrant JD, Lovrinic JH. *Bases of Hearing Science.* 3rd ed. Baltimore: Williams & Wilkins; 1995.

Janik VM, Sayigh LS, Wells, RS. Signature whistle shape conveys identity information to bottlenose dolphins. *PNAS,* 103(21):8293–8297.

Small AM: *Elements of Hearing Science: A Programmed Text.* New York: John Wiley & Sons; 1978.

Speaks C. *Introduction to Sound: Acoustics for the Hearing and Speech Sciences.* 3rd ed. San Diego: Singular Publishing Group; 1999.

Yost WA. *Fundamentals of Hearing: An Introduction.* 4th ed. New York: Academic Press; 2000.

CHAPTER 3

Structure and Function of the Auditory System

CHAPTER OBJECTIVES

- To be able to identify basic anatomical landmarks of the outer ear, middle ear, inner ear, and auditory portions of the central nervous system;
- To understand the primary functions of the outer ear, middle ear, inner ear, and auditory portions of the central nervous system;
- To gain insight into how the primary functions of each portion of the auditory system are supported by underlying anatomy and physiology; and
- To understand some basic perceptual aspects of sound such as hearing threshold, loudness, pitch, and masking.

KEY TERMS AND DEFINITIONS

- **Auditory periphery:** The outer ear, middle ear, and inner ear, ending at the nerve fibers exiting the inner ear.
- **Auditory central nervous system:** The ascending and descending auditory pathways in the brainstem and cortex.
- **Tonotopic organization:** The systematic mapping of sound frequency to the place of maximum stimulation within the auditory system that begins in the cochlea and is preserved through the auditory cortex.
- **Transducer:** A device or system that converts one form of energy to another. The cochlea can be considered a mechanoelectrical transducer because it converts mechanical vibrations to electrical energy to stimulate the afferent nerve fibers leading to the brainstem.

Recall that the primary purpose of the communication chain is to support the transfer of thoughts, ideas, or emotions between two people, the sender and the receiver. Thus far, we have seen that the sender can translate the thought to be communicated into a code of sound sequences representing meaningful words and sentences in the language shared by these two individuals. How is this acoustic code converted into information that can be understood by the mind of the receiver or listener? The mind of the receiver makes use of neural electrical signals generated by the central nervous system. Thus, one of the primary functions of the auditory system is to convert the acoustic energy produced by the talker—human speech sounds—into neural energy that can be deciphered by the brain of the listener. This process is the central topic of this chapter.

This chapter is divided into three main sections. The first two deal with the anatomy, physiology, and functional significance of the peripheral and central sections of the auditory system. The peripheral portion of the auditory system is defined here as the structures from the outer ear through the auditory nerve. The auditory portions of the central nervous system begin at the cochlear nucleus and end at the auditory centers of the cortex. The third section of this chapter details some fundamental aspects of the perception of sound.

PERIPHERAL AUDITORY SYSTEM

Figure 3.1 shows a cross-section of the **auditory periphery**. This portion of the auditory system is usually further subdivided into the outer ear, middle ear, and inner ear.

Outer Ear

The outer ear consists of two primary components: the pinna and the ear canal. The pinna is the most visible portion of the ear, which extends laterally from the side of the head. It is composed of cartilage and skin. The ear canal is the long, narrow canal leading to the eardrum (or tympanic membrane). The eardrum represents the boundary between the outer ear and the middle ear. The entrance to this canal is called the external auditory meatus. The deep bowl-like portion of the pinna adjacent to the external auditory meatus is known as the concha.

The outer ear serves a variety of functions. First, the long (2.5-cm), narrow (5- to 7-mm) canal makes the more delicate middle and inner ear less accessible to foreign objects. The outer third of the canal is composed of skin and

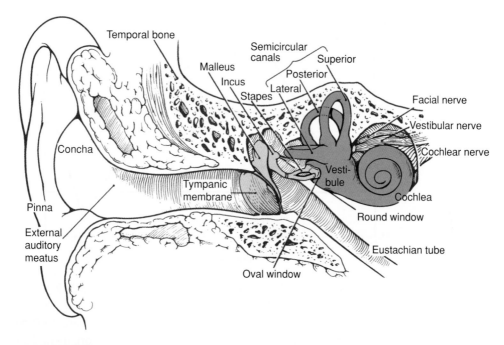

FIGURE 3.1 A cross-section of the peripheral portion of the auditory system revealing some of the anatomic details of the outer, middle, and inner ear. (Adapted from Kessel RG, Kardon RH. *Tissues and Organs: A Text-Atlas of Scanning Electron Microscopy.* San Francisco: WH Freeman; 1979, with permission.)

cartilage lined with glands and hairs. These glands, known as ceruminous glands, secrete a substance that potential intruders, such as insects, find terribly noxious. So both the long, narrow, tortuous path of the canal and the secretions of these glands serve to protect the remaining portions of the peripheral auditory system.

Second, the various air-filled cavities composing the outer ear, the two most prominent being the concha and the ear canal, have a natural or resonant frequency to which they respond best. This is true of all air-filled cavities and tubes. For an adult, the resonant frequency of the ear canal is approximately 2,500 Hz, whereas that of the concha is roughly 5,000 Hz. The resonance of each of these cavities is such that each structure increases the sound pressure at its resonant frequency by approximately 10 to 12 dB. This gain or increase in sound pressure provided by the outer ear can best be illustrated by considering the following hypothetical experiment.

Let us begin the experiment by using two tiny microphones. One microphone will be placed just outside (lateral to) the concha, and the other will be

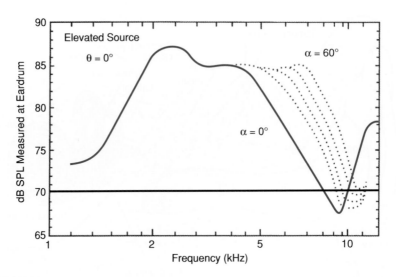

FIGURE 3.2 The response of the head, outer ear, and ear canal for various angles of elevation (a) of the sound source. Zero degrees corresponds to a sound source at eye level and straight ahead (0 degrees azimuth, 0 degrees elevation), whereas 60 degrees represents a source located straight ahead but at a higher elevation. If the listener's head and outer ear had no influence on the sound level measured at the eardrum, a flat line at 70 dB SPL would result. This figure illustrates the amplification of high-frequency sound by the outer ear and the way that this amplification pattern changes with elevation of the sound source. (Adapted from Shaw EAG. The external ear. In: Keidel WD, Neff WD, eds. *Handbook of Sensory Physiology,* vol 1. New York: Springer Verlag; 1974:463, with permission.)

positioned very carefully inside the ear canal to rest alongside the eardrum. Now if we present a series of sinusoidal sound waves, or pure tones, of different frequencies, which all measure 70 dB SPL at the microphone just outside the concha, and if we read the sound pressure levels measured with the other microphone near the eardrum, we will obtain results like those shown by the solid line in Figure 3.2. Notice that, at frequencies less than approximately 1,400 Hz, the microphone that is located near the eardrum measures sound levels of approximately 73 dB SPL. This is only 3 dB higher than the sound level just outside the outer ear. Consequently, the outer ear exerts little effect on the intensity of low-frequency sound. As the frequency of the sound is increased, however, the intensity of the sound measured at the eardrum increases to levels considerably above 70 dB SPL. The maximum sound level at the eardrum is reached at approximately 2,500 Hz and corresponds to a value of approximately 87 dB SPL. Thus, when sound waves having a frequency of

2,500 Hz enter the outer ear, their sound pressure levels are increased by 17 dB by the time they strike the eardrum. The function drawn with a solid line in Figure 3.2 illustrates the role that the outer ear serves as a resonator or amplifier of high-frequency sounds. The function shown is for the entire outer ear. Experiments similar to the one just described can be conducted to isolate the contribution of various cavities to the resonance of the total outer ear system. Again, the results of such experiments suggest that the two primary structures contributing to the resonance of the outer ear are the concha and the ear canal.

The resonance of the outer ear, which is represented by the solid line in Figure 3.2, was obtained with a sound source located directly in front of the subject at eye level. If the sound source is elevated by various amounts, a different resonance curve is obtained. Specifically, the notch or dip in the solid function that is located at 10 kHz in Figure 3.2 moves to a higher frequency and the peak of the resonant curve broadens to encompass a wider range of frequencies as the sound source is increased in elevation. This is illustrated in Figure 3.2 by the dotted lines. Each dotted line represents a different angle of elevation. An elevation of 0 degrees corresponds to eye level, whereas a 90-degree elevation would position the sound source directly overhead. The response of the outer ear changes as the elevation of the sound source changes. This results from the angle at which the incident sound wave strikes the various cavities of the outer ear. The result is that a code for sound elevation is provided by the outer ear. This code is the amplitude spectrum of the sound, especially above 3000 Hz, that strikes the eardrum. Thus, the outer ear plays an important role in the perception of the elevation of a sound source.

Finally, the outer ear also assists in another aspect of the localization of a sound source. The orientation of the pinnae is such that the pinnae collect sound more efficiently from sound sources located in front of the listener than from sources originating behind the listener. The attenuation of sound waves originating from behind the listener assists in the front/back localization of sound. This is especially true for high-frequency sounds (i.e., sounds with short wavelengths).

In summary, the outer ear serves four primary functions. First, it protects the more delicate middle and inner ears from foreign bodies. Second, it boosts or amplifies high-frequency sounds. Third, the outer ear provides the primary cue for the determination of the elevation of a sound's source. Fourth, the outer ear assists in distinguishing sounds that arise from in front of the listener from those that arise from behind the listener.

Middle Ear

The middle ear consists of a small (2-cm^3) air-filled cavity lined with a mucous membrane. It forms the link between the air-filled outer ear and the fluid-filled inner ear (Fig. 3.1). This link is accomplished mechanically via three tiny bones, the ossicles. The lateral-most ossicle is the malleus. The malleus is in contact with the eardrum or tympanic membrane. At the other end of the outer ear/inner ear link is the smallest, medial-most ossicle, the stapes. The broad base of the stapes, known as the footplate, rests in a membranous covering of the fluid-filled inner ear referred to as the oval window. The middle ossicle in the link, sandwiched between the malleus and stapes, is the incus. The ossicles are suspended loosely within the middle ear by ligaments extending from the anterior and posterior walls of the cavity.

We have mentioned that the middle ear cavity is air-filled. The air filling the cavity is supplied via a tube that connects the middle ear to the upper part of the throat, or the nasopharynx. This tube, known as the auditory tube or the eustachian tube, has one opening located along the bottom of the anterior wall of the middle ear cavity. The tube is normally closed but can be readily opened by yawning or swallowing. In adults, the eustachian tube assumes a slight downward orientation. This facilitates drainage of fluids from the middle ear cavity into the nasopharynx. Thus, the eustachian tube serves two primary purposes. First, it supplies air to the middle ear cavity and thereby enables an equalization of the air pressure on both sides of the eardrum. This is desirable for efficient vibration of the eardrum. Second, the eustachian tube permits the drainage of fluids from the middle ear into the nasopharynx.

What is the purpose of the elaborate link between the air-filled outer ear and the fluid-filled inner ear formed by the three ossicles? If the middle-ear cavity did not exist and the oval window on the cochlea was placed at the location of the eardrum, the acoustic energy would directly strike the fluid-filled inner ear and 99.9% of the energy in the impinging sound wave would be reflected away, with only 0.1% transmitted through to the inner ear. This loss amounts to a decrease in sound level of approximately 30 dB. Consequently, if such an arrangement existed, there would be a considerable loss of sound energy.

The middle ear compensates for this loss of sound energy when going from air to a fluid medium through two primary mechanisms. The first of these, the areal ratio (ratio of the areas) of the tympanic membrane to the footplate of the stapes, accounts for the largest portion of the compensation. The second mechanism, referred as a lever action of the ossicle, makes a very small contribution to the recovery of sound energy and is not considered further in this text. Regarding the areal ratio, the effective area of the tympanic membrane (i.e., the area involved directly in the mechanical link between the outer ear and inner ear) is approximately 55 mm^2. The corresponding area of the stapes footplate is 3.2 mm^2. Pressure (p) may be defined in terms of force (F) per unit area (A): $p = F/A$. If the force applied at the eardrum is the same as that reaching the stapes footplate, then the pressure at the smaller footplate must be greater than that at the larger eardrum. As an analogy, consider water being forced through a hose. If the area of the opening at the far end of the hose is the same as that of the faucet to which it is connected, the water will exit the hose under the same water pressure as it would at the faucet. If a nozzle is now attached to the far end of the hose and it is adjusted to decrease the size of the opening at that end of the hose, the water pressure at that end will be increased in proportion to the degree of constriction produced by the nozzle. The smaller the opening, the greater the water pressure at the nozzle (and the farther the water will be ejected from the nozzle). Applying the same force that exists at the faucet to push the water through a smaller opening created by the nozzle has increased the water pressure at the nozzle. Another analogy explaining the pressure gain associated with areal ratios is one that explains why carpentry nails have a broad head and sharp, narrow point (Vignette 3.1).

The middle ear system, primarily through the difference in area between the eardrum and the stapes footplate, compensates for much of the loss of sound energy that would result if the airborne sound waves impinged directly on the fluid-filled inner ear. Approximately 25 to 27 dB of the estimated 30-dB loss has been compensated for by the middle ear. The ability of the middle ear system to amplify or boost the sound pressure depends on signal frequency. Specifically, little pressure amplification occurs for frequencies below 100 Hz or above 2,000 to 2,500 Hz. Recall, however, that the outer ear amplified sound energy by 20 dB for frequencies from 2,000 to 5,000 Hz. Thus, taken together, the portion of the auditory system peripheral to the stapes footplate increases sound pressure by 20 to 25 dB in a range of approximately 100 to 5,000 Hz. This range of frequencies happens to correspond to the range of frequencies in human speech that are most important for communication. As is noted later in this chapter, a decrease of 10 dB in sound level for moderate-intensity sounds, such as conversational speech, corresponds to a halving of loudness. Without the amplification of sound waves provided by the outer and middle ears, conversational speech produced by the talker would sound like soft speech or whispered speech to the listener and effective communication would be jeopardized.

Another less obvious function of the middle ear also involves the outer ear/inner ear link formed by the ossicles. Because of the presence of this mechanical link, the preferred pathway for sound vibrations striking the eardrum will be along the chain formed by the three ossicles. Sound energy, therefore, will be routed directly to the oval window. There is another membranous window of the inner ear that also lies along the inner or medial wall of the middle ear cavity. This structure is known as the round window (Fig. 3.1). For the inner ear to be stimulated appropriately by the vibrations of the sound waves, it is important that the oval window and round window not be displaced

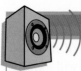

VIGNETTE 3.1 CONCEPTUAL DEMO

AN ANALOGY FOR PRESSURE

The common carpentry nail provides an illustration of the pressure amplification that occurs when the same force is applied over both a larger and smaller surface area. As shown in the figure, the head of the nail has a greater surface area than the narrow point of the nail. When force is applied to the broader head of the nail with a hammer, that same force is channeled through to the narrow point of the nail. However, because the area of the narrow point at the end of the nail is approximately 10 times smaller than the area at the head of the nail, the pressure applied at the narrow point is 10 times greater. (Recall that pressure is equal to force per unit area or Pressure = Force/Area.) The increased pressure at the point of the nail enables it to better penetrate the material (wood, for example) into which it is being driven. There are, of course, other practical factors affecting the design of the common carpentry nail (for example, the broader head also makes it easier to strike and to remove), but the resulting pressure amplification is one of the key elements in the design and represents a nice analogy to the pressure amplification achieved by the areal ratio of the tympanic membrane and stapes footplate in the middle ear.

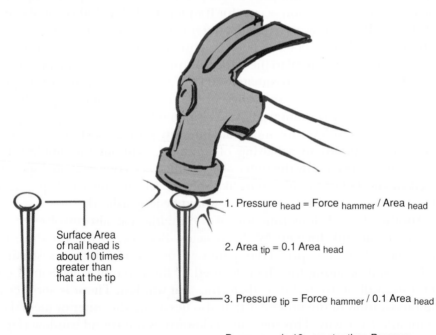

Surface Area of nail head is about 10 times greater than that at the tip

1. Pressure $_{head}$ = Force $_{hammer}$ / Area $_{head}$

2. Area $_{tip}$ = 0.1 Area $_{head}$

3. Pressure $_{tip}$ = Force $_{hammer}$ / 0.1 Area $_{head}$

Pressure $_{tip}$ is 10x greater than Pressure $_{head}$

in the same direction simultaneously. This situation would arise frequently, however, if the sound wave impinged directly on the medial wall of the middle ear cavity where both the oval window and the round window are located. Thus, routing the vibrations of the eardrum directly to the oval window via the ossicles assures appropriate stimulation of the inner ear.

Inner Ear

The inner ear is a complex structure that resides deep within a very dense portion of the skull known as the petrous portion of the temporal bone. Because of the complexity of this structure, it is often referred to as a labyrinth. The inner ear consists of a bony outer casing, the osseous labyrinth. Within this bony structure is the membranous labyrinth that contains the actual sensory structures. The osseous labyrinth, as shown in Figure 3.3, can be divided into three major sections: the *semicircular canals* (*superior, lateral,* and *posterior*), the *vestibule,* and the *cochlea.* The first two sections house the sensory organs for the vestibular system. The vestibular system assists in maintaining balance and posture. The focus here, however, will be placed on the remaining portion of the osseous inner ear, the cochlea. It is the cochlea that contains the sensory organ for hearing. The coiled, snail-shaped cochlea has approximately 2.75 turns in human beings. The largest turn is called the basal turn, and the smallest turn at the top of the cochlea is referred to as the apical turn. Two additional

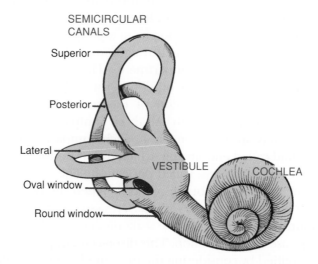

FIGURE 3.3 Illustration of the osseous labyrinth and its landmarks. (Adapted from Durrant JD, Lovrinic JH. *Bases of Hearing Science.* 2nd ed. Baltimore: Williams & Wilkins; 1984:98, with permission.)

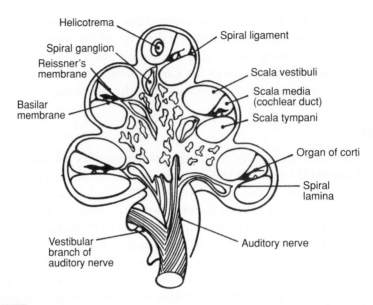

FIGURE 3.4 Modiolar cross-section of the cochlea illustrating the scalae through each of the turns. (Adapted from Zemlin WR. *Speech and Hearing Science: Anatomy and Physiology.* 2nd ed. Englewood Cliffs, NJ: Prentice-Hall; 1988:464, with permission.)

anatomic landmarks of the inner ear depicted in Figure 3.3 are the *oval window* and the *round window*. Recall that the footplate of the stapes, the medial-most bone of the three ossicles in the middle ear, is attached to the oval window.

The cochlea is cut in cross-section from top (apex) to bottom (base) in Figure 3.4. The winding channel running throughout the bony snail-shaped structure is further subdivided into three compartments. The middle compartment, the *scala media*, is sandwiched between the other two, the scala tympani and scala vestibuli. The scala media is a cross-section of the membranous labyrinth that runs throughout the osseous labyrinth. All three compartments are filled with fluid, although the fluids are not identical in each compartment. The scala media is filled with a fluid called endolymph, which differs considerably from the fluid in the other two compartments, called perilymph. The *scala media* houses the sensory organ for hearing, the organ of Corti. When the oval window vibrates as a consequence of vibration of the ossicles, a pressure wave is established within the fluid-filled inner ear that causes the scala media, and the structures within it, to move in response to the vibration. This displacement pattern for the scala media is usually simplified by considering the motion of just one of the partitions forming the scala media, the *basilar membrane* (Fig. 3.4). Although the displacement pattern of the basilar membrane is depicted, it should be noted that the entire fluid-filled scala media is undergoing similar displacement.

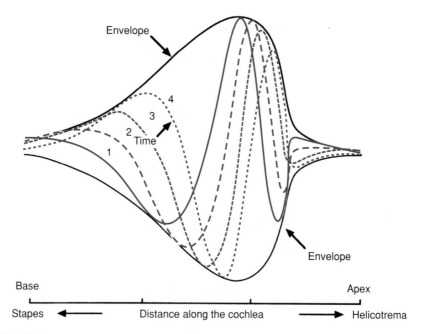

Base

Apex

Stapes ⟵   Distance along the cochlea   ⟶ Helicotrema

FIGURE 3.5 Illustration of the traveling wave pattern at four instants in time in response to a mid-frequency sound. The *thin solid lines* connect the maximum and minimum displacements at each location along the cochlea and for each instant in time. These lines represent the envelope of the displacement patterns. (Adapted from von Bekesy G. *Experiments in Hearing.* New York: McGraw-Hill; 1960:462.)

Figure 3.5 illustrates the displacement pattern of the basilar membrane at four successive instants in time. When this displacement pattern is visualized directly, the wave established along the basilar membrane is seen moving or traveling from the base to the apex. The displacement pattern increases gradually in amplitude as it progresses from the base toward the apex until it reaches a point of maximum displacement. At that point, the amplitude of displacement decreases abruptly. The thin solid line connecting the amplitude peaks at various locations for these four instants in time describes the displacement envelope. The envelope pattern is symmetrical in that the same pattern superimposed on the positive peaks can be flipped upside down and used to describe the negative peaks. As a result, only the positive or upper half of the envelope describing maximum displacement is usually displayed.

Figure 3.6 displays the envelopes of the displacement pattern of the basilar membrane that have been observed for different stimulus frequencies. Note that as the frequency of the stimulus increases, the peak of the displacement pattern moves in a basal direction closer to the stapes footplate. At low frequencies,

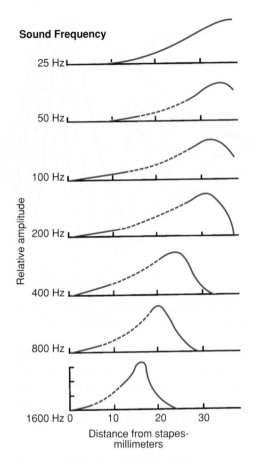

FIGURE 3.6 Envelopes of traveling wave displacement patterns illustrated for different stimulus frequencies. Notice that low frequencies (*top*) produce a maximum displacement of the basilar membrane in the apex (farthest distance from the stapes), whereas higher frequencies (*bottom*) produce maximum displacement in the basal portion of the cochlea (nearer to the stapes). (Adapted from von Bekesy G. *Experiments in Hearing.* New York: McGraw-Hill; 1960:448, with permission.)

virtually the entire membrane undergoes some degree of displacement. As stimulus frequency increases, a more restricted region of the basilar membrane undergoes displacement. Thus, the cochlea is performing a crude frequency analysis of the incoming sound. In general, for all but very low frequencies (≤50 Hz), the place of maximum displacement within the cochlea is associated with the frequency of an acoustic stimulus. The frequency of the acoustic stimulus striking the eardrum and displacing the stapes footplate will be analyzed or distinguished from sounds of different frequency by the location of the displacement pattern along the basilar membrane. This precise mapping of sound frequency to place of

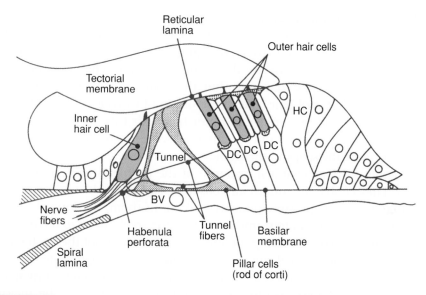

FIGURE 3.7 Detailed cross-section of the organ of Corti. *BV,* basilar vessel; *DC,* Deiter cell; *HC,* Hensen cell. (Adapted from Pickles JO. *An Introduction to the Physiology of Hearing.* 2nd ed. London: Academic Press; 1988:29.)

maximum mechanical activity in the cochlea is referred to as **tonotopic organization** (*tono* = frequency; *topic* = place; *tonotopic* = mapping of frequency to place of stimulation). Tonotopic organization is an important property of the auditory system, one that begins in the cochlea and is preserved to the auditory cortex, and forms the basis for viable code for sound frequency.

A more detailed picture of the structures within the scala media is provided in Figure 3.7. The sensory organ of hearing, the organ of Corti, is seen to rest on top of the basilar membrane. The organ of Corti contains several thousand sensory receptor cells called *hair cells.* Each hair cell has several tiny hairs or cilia protruding from the top of the cell. As shown in Figure 3.7, there are two types of hair cells within the organ of Corti: inner hair cells and outer hair cells. Approximately 90% to 95% of the auditory nerve fibers that carry information to the brain make contact with the inner hair cells. The outer hair cells are much greater in number, but do not have as many nerve-fiber connections to the upper portions of the auditory system (only 5% to 10% of nerve fibers connect to the outer hair cells). One of the critical functions of the hair cells in the organ of Corti is the conversion (**transducer** function) of mechanical energy from the middle-ear vibration to electrical energy that stimulates the connecting nerve fibers. As noted previously, this is a critical link in the communication chain in converting the acoustic signal from the sender to a neural electrical signal that can be deciphered by the brain of the receiver. The conversion takes place within the inner ear in the organ of Corti. Intact inner and outer hair cells are needed for this conversion to take place. As we will see later, many agents—such as noise, genetic disorders, or aging—can harm or destroy these hair cells and cause a breakdown in the communication chain. Although exciting research is underway that may alter this statement in the near future, at the moment, such loss of hair cells in the organ of Corti is irreversible.

If only a small percentage of outer hair cells (5% to 10%) are actually connected to the brain, what purpose do they serve? A complete answer to this question is beyond the scope of this book. Suffice it to say that the outer hair cells serve to augment the mechanical response of the cochlea when stimulated by vibrations. They enable the inner hair cells to be stimulated by much lower sound levels than would be possible otherwise. Without them, the inner hair cells would not be able to respond to sound levels lower than about 50 to 60 dB SPL. In addition, in the course of altering the mechanical response of the cochlea for incoming sound or mechanical vibration, the outer hair cells generate their own vibrations that can be recorded as sounds in the ear canal using a tiny microphone. These sounds, known as otoacoustic emissions (OAEs) can be measured and their presence can be used to verify a normal functioning cochlea (Vignette 3.2).

The two primary functions of the auditory portion of the inner ear can be summarized as follows. First, the inner ear performs a frequency analysis on incoming sounds so that different frequencies stimulate different regions of the inner ear (i.e., tonotopic organization). Second, mechanical vibration is amplified and converted into electrical energy by the hair cells. The hair cells are frequently referred to as mechanoelectrical transducers. That is, cells that convert mechanical energy (vibration) into electrical energy that leads to the generation of electrical activity in the auditory nerve.

Auditory Nerve

The electrical potentials generated by auditory nerve fibers are called all-or-none action potentials because they do not vary in amplitude when activated. If the nerve fibers fire, they always fire to the same degree, reaching 100% amplitude. The action potentials, moreover, are very short-lived events, typically requiring less than 1 to 2 ms to rise in amplitude to maximum potential and return to resting state. For this reason, they are frequently referred to as *spikes*. Information is coded in the auditory portions of the central nervous system via patterns of neural spikes. For example, as the intensity of sound is increased, the rate at which an auditory nerve fiber fires also increases, although only over a limited range of variation in sound intensity.

By varying the intensity and frequency of the sound stimulus, it is possible to determine the frequency to which a given nerve fiber responds best; that is,

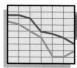

VIGNETTE 3.2   CLINICAL APPLICATIONS

Use of OAEs as a Screening Tool for Babies

The development of tools to measure OAEs clinically has led to many exciting applications. For the first time in the history of clinical audiology, a tool was made available that measured the integrity of the sensory receptors in the generally inaccessible inner ear.

One of the clinical applications explored and refined during the 1990s was the use of OAEs as a screening tool for hearing loss in infants. Some of the advantages associated with the use of OAEs for this application included the ability to record these responses without requiring the active participation of the infant, the ability to assess each ear separately, and the capability of evaluating a fairly broad range of frequencies. In addition, normal OAE responses would only be possible with normal outer, middle, and inner ears. The focus in OAE-based screening is clearly on the auditory periphery. Problems localized to any of these sections of the auditory periphery, moreover, are most amenable to intervention, either medical (for outer and middle ears) or audiologic (in the form of hearing aids or other prosthetic devices for those with inner ear problems).

Many states have adopted legislation in recent years that requires that all infants be screened for hearing loss at birth (referred to as "universal screening"). Screening tools based on OAEs represent one of the most commonly used devices in universal newborn screening programs.

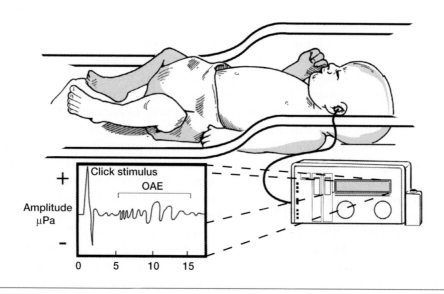

the frequency that requires the least amount of intensity to produce an increase in firing rate. This frequency is often referred to as the *best frequency* or *characteristic frequency* of the nerve fiber. Some nerve fibers have a low characteristic frequency and some have a high characteristic frequency. Fibers with high characteristic frequencies come from (inner) hair cells in the base of the cochlea, whereas those with low characteristic frequencies supply the apex. As the nerve fibers exit through the bony core of the cochlea on their way to the brainstem, they maintain an orderly arrangement. The bundle of nerve fibers composing the cochlear branch of the auditory nerve is organized so that fibers with high characteristic frequencies are located around the perimeter, whereas fibers with low characteristic frequencies make up the core of the cochlear nerve. Thus, the auditory nerve is organized, as is the basilar membrane, so that each characteristic frequency corresponds to a specific anatomical location or place. This mapping of the frequency of the sound wave to place of maximum activity within an anatomic structure is referred to as *tonotopic organization.* The neural place that responds to a particular sound stimulus provides the brain with important information regarding the frequency content of that sound.

Temporal or time-domain information is also coded by fibers of the auditory nerve. Consider, for example, the discharge pattern that occurs within a nerve fiber when that stimulus is a sinusoid that lies within the response area of the nerve fiber. The pattern of spikes that occurs under such conditions is illustrated in Figure 3.8. Note that when the single nerve fiber discharges, it always does so at essentially the same location on the stimulus waveform. In Figure 3.8, this happens to be the positive peak of the waveform. Notice also that it may not fire during every cycle of the stimulus waveform. Nonetheless, if one were to record the interval between successive spikes and examine the number of times each interval occurred, a histogram of the results would look like that shown in Figure 3.8. This histogram, known simply as an interval histogram, indicates that the most frequent interspike interval corresponds to the period of the waveform. All other peaks in the histogram occur at integer multiples of the period. Thus, the nerve fiber is able to encode the period of the waveform. This holds true for nerve fibers with characteristic frequencies less than approximately 5,000 Hz. As discussed in Chapter 2, if we know the period of a sinusoidal waveform, we know its frequency ($f = 1/T$). Hence, the nerve fibers responding in the manner depicted in Figure 3.8 could code the frequency of the acoustic stimulus according to the timing of discharges. For frequencies up to 5,000 Hz, the neural firing is synchronized to the sound stimulus, as in Figure 3.8A. By combining synchronized firings for several nerve fibers, it is possible to encode the period of sounds up to 5,000 Hz in frequency. This type of frequency coding may be useful for a wide variety of sounds, including the coding of the fundamental frequency for complex sounds like vowels or musical notes.

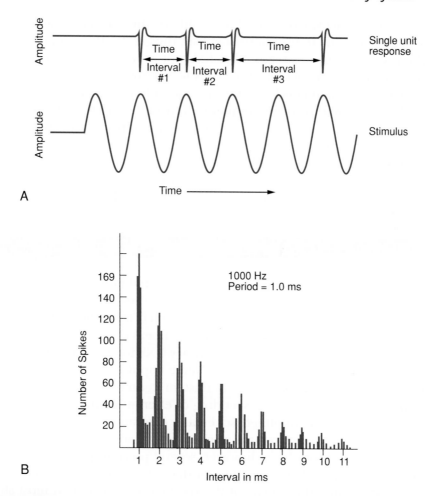

FIGURE 3.8   A, Illustration of the synchronization of nerve fiber firings to the stimulus waveform. Note that the nerve fiber always fires at the same point of the waveform, although it may not fire every cycle. The intervals between successive firings of the nerve fiber can be measured and stored for later analysis. B, A histogram of the intervals measured in (A), referred to as interspike intervals. An interval of 1 ms was the most frequently occurring interval, having occurred approximately 180 times. This corresponds to the period of the waveform in (A).

The electrical activity of the auditory nerve can also be recorded from more remote locations. In this case, however, the action potentials are not being measured from single nerve fibers. Recorded electrical activity under these circumstances represents the composite response from a large number of nerve fibers. For this reason, this composite electrical response is referred to frequently as the *whole-nerve action potential*. Because the whole-nerve action potential represents the summed activity of several nerve fibers, the greater the number of fibers that can be made to fire simultaneously, the greater the summed amplitude of the response. For this reason, brief abrupt acoustic signals, such as clicks, are used as stimuli. A click stimulus rises to maximum amplitude in a very short period of time and lasts for a short period of time (e.g., less than 1 ms). A click is also comprised of many frequencies from 0 to 10,000 Hz. As such, a click stimulus stimulates nerve fibers from the high-frequency basal region to the low-frequency apical region of the cochlea and does so almost instantaneously. With such a large number of nerve fibers firing nearly simultaneously, the electrical activity generated by the cochlea's nerve fibers can be measured with recording electrodes in the ear canal or on the scalp.

AUDITORY CENTRAL NERVOUS SYSTEM

Once the action potentials have been generated in the cochlear branch of the auditory nerve, the electrical activity progresses up toward the cortex. This network of nerve fibers is frequently referred to as the **auditory central nervous system** (auditory CNS). The nerve fibers that carry information in the form of action potentials up the auditory CNS toward the cortex form part of the ascending or afferent pathways. Nerve impulses can also be sent toward the periphery from the cortex or brainstem centers. The fibers carrying such information compose the descending or efferent pathways.

Figure 3.9 is a simplified schematic diagram of the ascending auditory CNS. All nerve fibers from the cochlea terminate at the cochlear nucleus on the same side. From here, however, several possible paths are available. The majority of nerve fibers cross over or decussate at some point along the auditory CNS, so that the activity of the right ear is represented most strongly on the left side of the cortex and vice versa. The crossover, however, is not complete. From the superior olives through the cortex, activity from both ears is represented on each side. In fact, this represents one of the key functions of the auditory CNS: combining or integrating the neural information from both ears. This is referred to as binaural (or "two-ear") processing and is critical for some aspects of sound perception, including our ability to locate sounds in space. All ascending fibers terminate in the medial geniculate body before ascending to the cortex. Thus, all ascending fibers within the brainstem portion of the auditory CNS synapse at the cochlear nucleus and at the medial geniculate body, taking one of several paths between these two points, with many paths having additional intervening nerve fibers. Vignette 3.3 describes measurement of the auditory brainstem response and its correlation with anatomic structure.

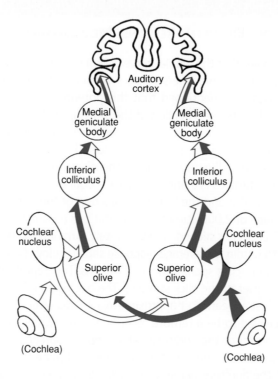

FIGURE 3.9 The ascending pathways of the auditory central nervous system. The *blue arrows* represent input from the right ear; the *white arrows* represent input from the left ear. (Adapted from Yost WA, Nielsen DW. *Fundamentals of Hearing: An Introduction.* 2nd ed. New York: Holt, Rinehart, & Winston; 1985:98, with permission.)

We have already reviewed the simple coding of information available in the responses of the auditory nerve fibers. The mapping of frequency to place within the cochlea, for example, was preserved in the responses of the nerve fibers such that fibers having high characteristic frequencies originated from the high-frequency base of the cochlea. The period of the waveform could also be coded for stimulus frequencies less than 5,000 Hz. In addition, the intensity of the stimulus is coded over a limited range (30 to 40 dB) by the discharge rate of the fiber. At the level of the cochlear nucleus, it is already apparent that the ascending auditory pathway begins processing information by converting this fairly simple code into more complex codes. The coding of timing information, for example, is much more complex in the cochlear nucleus. In addition, some nerve fibers within the cochlear nucleus have a much broader range of intensities (up to 100 dB) over which the discharge rate increases steadily with sound intensity. As one probes nerve fibers at various centers within the auditory CNS, a tremendous diversity of responses is evident.

Auditory Brainstem Response Measurements

It was mentioned earlier that the whole-nerve action potential represented the summed response of many single nerve fibers firing synchronously in response to an abrupt acoustic signal. It was also mentioned that this potential could be recorded remotely from the ear canal. The left-hand portion of the drawing that accompanies this vignette shows a patient with electrodes pasted to the skin of the forehead, the top of the head (vertex), and the area behind the pinna (the mastoid prominence). The tracing in the right-hand portion of this illustration shows the electrical activity recorded from the patient. The acoustic stimulus is a brief click that produces synchronized responses from nerve fibers in the cochlea and the brainstem portion of the auditory CNS. The tracing represents the average of 2,000 stimulus presentations presented at a moderate intensity at a rate of 11 clicks per second. Approximately 3 minutes is required to present all 2,000 stimuli and to obtain the average response shown below. Note that the time scale for the x axis of the tracing spans from 0 to 10 ms. This represents a 10-ms interval beginning with the onset of the click stimulus. The tracing shows several distinct bumps or waves, with the first appearing at approximately 1.5 ms after stimulus onset. This first wave, wave I, is believed to be a remote recording of the whole-nerve action potential from the closest portion of the auditory nerve. Approximately 1 ms later, 2.5 ms after stimulus onset, wave II is observed. This wave is believed to be the response of the more distant portion of the auditory nerve. One millisecond later, the electrical activity has traveled to the next center in the brainstem, the cochlear nucleus, and produces the response recorded as wave III. Wave IV represents the activity of the superior olivary complex. Wave V represents the response of the lateral lemniscus, a structure lying between the superior olives and the inferior colliculus. Waves VI and VII (the two unlabeled bumps after wave V) represent the response of the latter brainstem structure.

The response shown in the right-hand tracing is known as an auditory brainstem response (ABR). It has proven very useful in a wide variety of clinical applications, from assessment of the functional integrity of the peripheral and brainstem portions of the ascending auditory CNS to assessment of hearing in infants or difficult-to-test patients.

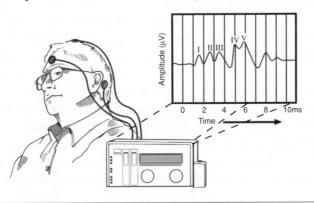

Despite this increasing anatomic and physiologic complexity, one thing that appears to be preserved throughout the auditory CNS is tonotopic organization. At each brainstem center and within the auditory portions of the cortex, there is an orderly mapping of frequency to place. This can be demonstrated by measuring the characteristic frequency of nerve fibers encountered at various locations within a given brainstem center or within the cortex.

Another principle underlying the auditory CNS is that of redundancy. That is, information represented in the neural code from one ear has multiple representations at various locations within the auditory system. Every auditory nerve fiber, for example, splits into two fibers before entering the cochlear nucleus, with each branch supplying a different region of the cochlear nucleus. In addition, from the superior olives through the auditory areas of the cortex, information from both ears is represented at each location in the auditory CNS. This redundancy in the auditory CNS helps to protect the communication chain against breakdowns. A lesion, such as a tumor, on one side of the brainstem, for example, will not necessarily prevent information from both ears reaching the auditory portions of the cortex.

Perception of Sound

The basic structure and some key aspects of the physiologic function of the auditory system have been reviewed; the remainder of this chapter reviews some fundamental aspects of the perception of sound by humans. We have examined the acoustics involved in the generation and propagation of a sound wave and have reviewed its conversion into a complex neural code. This code of incoming sensory information can influence the behavior of a human subject, whether the sound is the loud whistle of an oncoming train or the soft voice of a precocious toddler.

The lowest sound pressure that can be reliably heard by a human listener is referred to as the listener's hearing threshold. The results obtained from the measurement of hearing thresholds at various frequencies are depicted in Figure 3.10. Note that the sound pressure level that is just detectable varies with frequency, especially below 500 Hz and above 8,000 Hz. The range of audibility of the normal-hearing human ear is described frequently as 20 to 20,000 Hz. Acoustic signals at frequencies above or below this range typically cannot be heard by the normal human ear.

The phenomenon of masking has also been studied in detail. Masking refers to the ability of one acoustic signal to obscure the presence of another acoustic signal so that it cannot be detected. A whisper might be audible, for example, in a quiet environment. In a noisy industrial environment, however, such a weak acoustic signal would be masked by the more intense factory noise.

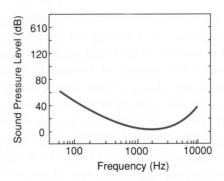

FIGURE 3.10   Average normal threshold sound pressure level plotted as a function of frequency for binaural (two-ear) listening in a free field. (Adapted from Sivian LJ, White SD. Minimum audible pressure and minimum audible field. *J Acoust Soc Amer.* 1933;4:288–321.)

Masking is used clinically to aid the audiologist in the diagnosis of hearing difficulties, as will be discussed in more detail in a subsequent chapter.

Loudness is clearly one of the more salient perceptual features of a sound and it also has considerable clinical importance. As noted previously, there are many agents that can destroy the outer hair cells of the cochlea, including high-intensity noise and aging. When this occurs, the listener loses the ability to hear soft sounds in the frequency regions associated with the loss of hair cells. For example, if the hair cell loss was in the basal portion of the cochlea, then the listener would have difficulty hearing low-intensity, high-frequency sounds. The loudness of high-intensity sounds, however, is not impacted much by the loss of outer hair cells and this same individual would hear loud sounds normally. As will be noted later, this represents a potential "break" in the communication chain with input to the higher centers distorted by a loss of hair cells in the cochlea. In this particular case of loss of outer hair cells only, the conventional hearing aid represents a reasonable approach to the repair of the communication chain.

Pitch is another very salient perceptual feature of sound. In general, pitch is the perceptual correlate of sound frequency. We have already seen that the auditory system is capable of coding sound frequency via place of stimulation (tonotopic organization) and timing information, such as the period of the waveform. This perceptual pitch information can aid in the identification of specific talker voices or fundamental frequencies, as well as elements of the speech sounds produced by a talker, such as the formant frequencies of vowels. It is generally believed that the pitch associated with sound frequencies below 50 Hz are mediated exclusively by timing information because, as noted previously, tonotopic organization breaks down at these very low frequencies. On the other hand, because timing information breaks down above 5,000 Hz due to the loss of synchronous neural firing of the auditory nerve, place coding predominates at these higher frequencies. For frequencies between 50 and 5,000 Hz, both place-based and timing-based codes for sound frequency may underlie the perceived pitch. An overview of some interesting early research on timing-based and place-based codes for pitch perception is provided in Vignette 3.4.

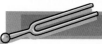

VIGNETTE 3.4   EXPERIMENT

PITCH PERCEPTION AND "THE CASE OF THE MISSING FUNDAMENTAL"

As noted, the pitch of a sound is often one of its most salient perceptual characteristics. Musicians and hearing scientists have been interested in how humans perceive pitch for centuries, but probably the greatest progress in our understanding of pitch perception occurred during the 20th century.

In the late 19th century, probably the most accepted theory of pitch perception was based on a "place principle" akin to tonotopic organization described previously in the discussion of basic auditory structure and function. Although many details of early

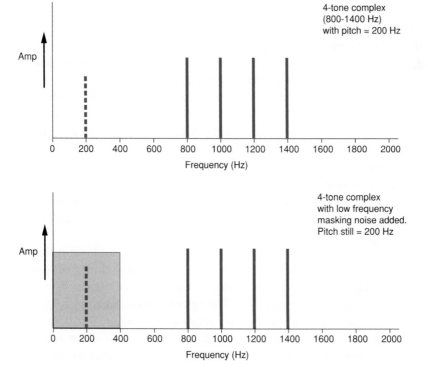

place-principle theories of pitch perception were incorrect, the basic premise that certain portions of the auditory system, especially the inner ear, were "tuned" to specific frequencies was correct. Basically, low-frequency pure tones produced a low pitch sensation and high-frequency pure tones produced a high pitch sensation because each frequency stimulated a different region or place within the inner ear.

In the late 19th and early 20th centuries, however, several researchers in the Netherlands produced a low-frequency pitch using sounds that were comprised of only higher frequencies. An example of the amplitude spectrum for one such sound is shown in the figure. Notice that this sound is comprised of pure tones at frequencies of 800, 1,000, 1,200, and 1,400 Hz. Yet, the pitch of this sound was judged to be 200 Hz by listeners. A frequency of 200 Hz would correspond to the fundamental frequency of these sounds with 800 Hz being the fourth harmonic of 200 Hz (i.e., 800 Hz = 4 × 200 Hz), 1,000 Hz being the fifth harmonic, 1,200 Hz being the sixth harmonic, and 1,400 Hz being the seventh harmonic of 200 Hz. For this reason, the pitch of such a series of pure tones is often referred to as the "missing fundamental."

Now, the place theorists simply argued that the equipment or the ear (the middle ear was believed to be the culprit at the time) generated a distortion product that corresponded to the 200-Hz frequency, and the listener's pitch perception was dominated by this low-frequency distortion tone. Therefore, the fundamental frequency (200 Hz) was not really missing after all. In this way, the results were entirely consistent with the place theory. The complex of four pure tones from 800 to 1,400 Hz generated a distortion product at 200 Hz; this 200-Hz distortion product stimulated the place associated with a 200-Hz pure tone yielding a corresponding pitch.

To counter this argument, the Dutch researchers conducted the following experiment. A low-frequency noise was introduced with enough acoustical energy below 400 Hz to mask low-frequency tones of moderate intensity (as demonstrated with a pure tone at 200 Hz, for example). The four pure tones from 800 to 1,400 Hz were played in this background of low-frequency noise, and a pitch of 200 Hz was again perceived. Basically, the low-frequency masking noise rendered the low-frequency region of the inner ear unusable, and yet, a low-frequency pitch was still perceived when the four tones from 800 to 1,400 Hz were presented. Clearly, the place theory could not account for these findings.

Recognizing the limitations of the place theory as a single explanation for the perception of pitch, hearing scientists began to focus on possible timing or "periodicity" cues present in the four-tone complex. Today, although several details of pitch perception remain unexplained, the majority of findings can be described by a "duplex" theory that relies on exclusive use of place cues above approximately 5,000 Hz (recall that synchronization of nerve fiber firing breaks down at frequencies above approximately 5,000 Hz, making timing or "periodicity" cues unavailable), exclusive use of timing cues for very low frequencies below approximately 50 Hz, and a combination of both periodicity and place cues for frequencies from 50 to 5,000 Hz.

Incidentally, there is a standardized scale of pitch sensation referred to as the Mel scale (no, not named after a famous scientist named "Mel" but derived from "melody"). A pure tone of 1,000 Hz at 40 dB SPL is said to have a pitch of 1,000 mels (as well as a loudness of 1 sone and a loudness level of 40 phons). A sound with a pitch judged to be twice as high as this standard would have a pitch of 2,000 mels, whereas one with half the pitch of the standard sound would be assigned a pitch value of 500 mels. Often, however, pitch is measured by matching the frequency of a pure tone to the perceived pitch of the sound under evaluation.

SUMMARY

In this chapter, we have seen how the acoustic information, serving as the link between the sender and the receiver in the communication chain, is encoded by the auditory system. Initially, the pressure fluctuations corresponding to the acoustic speech sounds are converted into mechanical vibrations of the middle ear and organ of Corti. These mechanical vibrations are converted to electrical signals by the organ of Corti and ultimately lead to the generation of electrical signals in the auditory nerve. The sensory input representing the acoustic speech stimulus is now in the "electrical language" of the brain and is subject to further processing by the auditory centers of the brainstem and cortex. This neural auditory information in the auditory cortex is then processed, as needed, by other centers of the brain, such as various language-processing centers, to make sense of the incoming sensory information. Impairments in the auditory periphery or auditory portions of the central nervous system can result in "breaks" in the communication chain, with degraded neural information reaching the higher centers of the auditory system. The identification of such impairments is the focus of the Chapter 4.

CHAPTER REVIEW QUESTIONS

1. What are the primary functions of the outer ear?
2. What is the primary function of the middle ear and what is the main anatomical feature that supports this function?
3. The Eustachian tube serves two main functions. What are they?
4. Define tonotopic organization. Where does it originate? Based on this anatomical organization, if an individual lost all inner and outer hair cells in the base of the cochlea, what sound frequencies would this person have difficulty hearing?
5. What is meant by the "transducer function" of the cochlea?
6. Frequency can be encoded by the auditory periphery using a placed-based code or a timing-based code. Explain what this means.
7. What structures represent the beginning and ending of the auditory central nervous system?
8. Aside from the initial letter in their spelling, what is the difference between "afferent" and "efferent" nerve fibers?
9. In very general terms, loudness and pitch can be considered to be the perceptual correlates of what two physical aspects of sound waves?

REFERENCES AND SUGGESTED READINGS

Durrant JD, Lovrinic JH. *Bases of Hearing Science.* 2nd ed. Baltimore: Williams & Wilkins; 1995.

Geisler CD. *From Sound to Synapse.* New York: Oxford University Press; 1998.

Gelfand SA. *Hearing: An Introduction to Psychological and Physiological Acoustics.* 3rd ed. New York: Marcel Dekker; 1997.

Hall JW. *Handbook of Auditory Evoked Responses.* Needham, MA: Allyn & Bacon; 1992.

Kidd J. Psychoacoustics. In Katz J, ed. *Handbook of Clinical Audiology.* 5th ed. Philadelphia: Lippincott Williams & Wilkins; 2002.

Möller AR. *Auditory Physiology.* New York: Academic Press; 1983.

Moore BCJ. *An Introduction to the Psychology of Hearing.* 4th ed. London: Academic Press; 1997.

Pickles JO. *An Introduction to the Physiology of Hearing.* 2nd ed. London: Academic Press; 1988.

Probst R, Lonsbury-Martin BL, Martin G. A review of otoacoustic emissions. *J Acoust Soc Amer.* 1991;89:2027–2067.

Shaw EAG. The external ear. In Keidel WD, Neff WD, eds. *Handbook of Sensory Physiology.* Vol. 1. New York: Springer Verlag; 1974: 455–490.

von Bekesy G. *Experiments in Hearing.* New York: McGraw-Hill; 1960.

Wever EG, Lawrence M. *Physiological Acoustics.* Princeton: Princeton University Press; 1954.

Yost WA. *Fundamentals of Hearing: An Introduction.* 4th ed. New York: Academic Press; 2000.

Zemlin WR. *Speech and Hearing Science: Anatomy and Physiology.* 2nd ed. Englewood Cliffs, NJ: Prentice-Hall; 1988.

Zwicker E, Fastl H. *Psychoacoustics.* 2nd ed. Berlin: Springer-Verlag; 1999.

CHAPTER 4

Auditory Disorders

CHAPTER OBJECTIVES

- To understand various classification systems for disorders of the auditory system;
- To appreciate the strong role played by genetics in many auditory disorders;
- To learn how otitis media develops and its potential consequences for communication; and
- To become familiar with several of the more prevalent or more severe disorders affecting the cochlea, and their consequences for communication.

KEY TERMS AND DEFINITIONS

- **Endogenous:** A trait or disorder that arises from the individual's genes.
- **Exogenous:** A trait or disorder that is not attributable to genetic causes.
- **Congenital:** A trait or disorder that is present at birth, but may or may not be of genetic origin.
- **Otitis media:** An inflammation of the mucosal lining of the middle-ear cavity that may include the accumulation of fluid in the cavity.
- **Presbycusis:** Loss of hearing that occurs with advancing age, especially beyond the age of 60 years.
- **Retrocochlear pathology:** A disease or disorder of the auditory system that impacts structures located from the auditory nerve through the auditory cortex (i.e., "beyond the cochlea").

A variety of disorders, both congenital and acquired, directly affect the auditory system and can result in breaks in the communication chain. These disorders can occur at the level of the external ear, the external auditory canal, the tympanic membrane, the middle ear space, the cochlea, the auditory central nervous system, or any combination of these sites. The following review offers a discussion of some of the more commonly seen disorders that can impair the auditory system.

CLASSIFICATION OF AUDITORY DISORDERS

All auditory disorders can be divided into two major classifications: **exogenous** or **endogenous.** Exogenous hearing disorders are those caused by inflammatory disease, toxicity, noise, accident, or injury that inflicts damage on any part of the auditory system. Endogenous conditions originate in the genetic characteristics of an individual. An endogenous auditory defect is transmitted from the parents to the child as an inherited trait. However, not all **congenital** hearing disorders (i.e., those present at birth) are hereditary, nor are all hereditary disorders congenital. For example, the child whose hearing mechanism is damaged in utero by maternal rubella is born with a hearing loss. This hearing loss is congenital but not hereditary. On the other hand, some hereditary defects of hearing may not manifest themselves until adulthood. A breakdown of the estimated percentage of individuals with exogenous and endogenous types of hearing loss is shown in Figure 4.1.

Genetic Transmission of Hearing Loss

As Figure 4.1 shows, hearing loss resulting from hereditary factors is thought to make up approximately 50% of all auditory disorders. It is estimated that there are more than 400 different genetic syndromes in which hearing loss is a regular or occasional feature (Table 4.1). This is referred to as *syndromic hearing loss* because it is one symptom of several comprising a genetic syndrome. In addition, there are at least 35 types of genetic deafness that are known to occur without any other associated anomalies. This is referred to as *nonsyndromic hearing loss*; hearing loss is the only symptom or feature of the genetic disorder. Of all cases of genetic hearing loss, about 20% to 30% are syndromic and 70% to 80% are nonsyndromic.

Whether occurring as one manifestation of a particular syndrome (group of signs/symptoms that characterize a disorder or condition) or with no other abnormalities, hereditary hearing loss is usually governed by the Mendelian laws of inheritance. According to these genetic laws, genetic traits may be

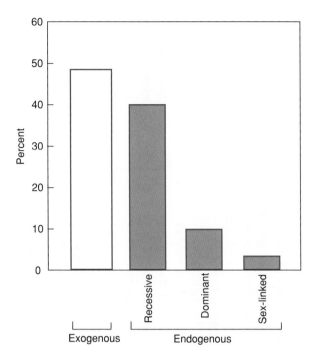

FIGURE 4.1 Percentage of individuals that exhibit exogenous and endogenous types of hearing loss.

dominant or recessive. Genes are located on the chromosomes and, with the exception of those genes that are located on the sex chromosomes of males, they come in pairs. One member of each gene pair (and the corresponding member of a chromosome pair) is inherited from each parent. Humans have 22 pairs of autosomes, or nonsex-determining chromosomes, and one pair of sex-determining chromosomes. The sex chromosome pair for females consists of two X chromosomes; for males, it consists of one X and one Y chromosome. In the process of human reproduction, each egg and each sperm cell carries one half of the chromosomes of each parent. When the egg is fertilized, the full complement of chromosomes is restored, so that half of a child's genes are from the mother and half are from the father.

Most genes are located in the nucleus of a cell, but genetic material can also be found in the cell's mitochondria. Mitochondria are transmitted to each of the offspring exclusively via the mother's egg. Some forms of genetic hearing loss have been associated with defects in the mitochondria. If the mother has such a genetic defect, she will pass the hearing loss to all of her offspring.

TABLE 4.1 Examples of Autosomal Dominant, Recessive, and Sex-Linked Syndromic Forms of Hereditary Hearing Loss

Mode of Transmission/ Disorder	Prevalence	Clinical Characteristics	Hearing Loss
Autosomal Dominant			
Waardenburg syndrome	1/4000; 3% of childhood hearing loss	Pigmentary anomalies (white forelock, blue irises, premature graying, partial albinism) cranio-facial anomalies—hyper-telorism, high nasal bridge, synophrys	20–50% exhibit SNHL depending on expres-sion of syndrome
Branchio-oto-renal syndrome	1/40,000; 2% of children with profound hearing loss	Branchial abnormalities—ear pits and tags, cysts and fistula; renal abnormalities	75% exhibit hearing loss; 30% conductive, 20% SNHL, 50% mixed
Treacher Collins syndrome	Unknown	Craniofacial anomalies: poorly developed malar bones, notching of eye-lids, malformations of the external ear or canal, micronathia, cleft palate	30% exhibit conductive hearing loss, SNHL may be present
Recessive			
Usher syndrome	3.5/100,000; 10% of childhood hearing loss	SNHL and retinitis pigmentosa	Type 1: congenital bilateral profound hearing loss and absent vestibular function; Type 2: moderate bilateral SNHL and normal vestibular function

			Type 3: progressive bilateral SNHL, variable vestibular dysfunction, found primarily in Norwegian population
Pendred syndrome	Unknown; 5% of congenital childhood hearing loss	Thyroid goiter and SNHL	Severe to profound SNHL, 15% may be progressive
Jervell and Lange-Neilsen syndrome	Unknown (rare)	SNHL and syncopal episodes	Profound bilateral SNHL
Sex-Linked			
Norrie syndrome	Unknown	SNHL, congenital or rapidly progressive blindness, pseudoglioma, opacification, and ocular degeneration	One third exhibit progressive SNHL beginning in 2nd or 3rd decade of life
Alport syndrome	Unknown (predilection for males)	SNHL and nephritis	Bilateral progressive SNHL

SNHL, sensorineural hearing loss.

Autosomal Dominant Inheritance

In autosomal dominant inheritance, the trait is carried from one generation to another. The term *autosomal* implies that the abnormal gene is not located on one of the two sex chromosomes. Typically, one parent exhibits the inherited trait, which may be transmitted to 50% of the offspring. This does not mean that half the children in a given family will necessarily be affected. Statistically, there is a 50% chance that any given child, whether male or female, will be affected (Vignette 4.1). Autosomal dominant inheritance is believed to account for approximately 20% of cases of genetically caused (endogenous) deafness. Because of the interaction of a number of genes, some traits may manifest themselves only partially; for example, only a very mild hearing loss may be observed despite a genetic structure indicating profound hearing loss.

Autosomal Recessive Inheritance

In contrast to autosomal dominant inheritance, both parents of a child with hearing loss of the autosomal recessive type are often clinically normal. Appearance of the trait in the offspring requires that an individual possess two similar abnormal genes, one from each parent. The parents themselves are often *heterozygous* carriers of a single abnormal recessive gene. This means that each carries two different genes, one normal and one abnormal with respect to a particular gene pair. Offspring carrying two of either the normal or the abnormal type of gene are termed *homozygotes*. Offspring may also be heterozygotes like their parents, carrying one of each gene type. If no abnormal gene is transmitted, the offspring is normal for that trait. If there is one abnormal gene, the child becomes a *carrier* for the trait. Finally, if two abnormal genes, one from each parent, are transmitted, the offspring is affected and becomes a homozygous carrier. The probability that heterozygote parents will bear an affected, homozygous child is 25% in each pregnancy on the basis that each child would inherit the abnormal gene from both the father (50% chance) and the mother (50% chance). Because the laws of probability permit this type of hearing loss to be transmitted without manifestation through several generations, the detection of the true origin is often quite difficult. Recessive genes account for the majority of cases of genetic hearing loss and can account for as much as 80% of childhood deafness.

X-Linked Inheritance

In the X-linked type of deafness, inherited traits are determined by genes located on the X chromosome. As noted earlier, normal females have two X chromosomes, whereas males possess one X and one Y chromosome. Sons

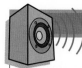

#5

ILLUSTRATION OF MENDELIAN LAW

For this demonstration, you will need two paper cups and five poker chips or checkers (three chips of one color and two of another). For the first illustration, select one chip of one color and three of the other color. We will assume that you have one white chip and three blue ones. Divide the four chips into two pairs, each pair representing a parent. The white chip represents a dominant gene for deafness. Whenever it is paired with another white chip or a blue chip, it dominates the trait for hearing, resulting in deafness in the person with the gene. In this example, we have one Deaf parent (one blue chip, one white chip) and one normal-hearing parent (two blue chips).

Each parent contributes one gene for hearing status to each offspring. When the Deaf parent contributes the gene for deafness (white chip), the offspring will always be Deaf. This is because the normal-hearing parent has only recessive genes for normal hearing (blue chips) to contribute to the offspring. Separate the white chip from the Deaf parent and slide it toward you. Slide each of the blue chips from the other parent toward you, one at a time. For both of these possible offspring, the child will be Deaf (a white chip paired with a blue one). Now return the chips to the parents and slide the blue chip from the Deaf parent close to you. Slide each of the blue chips from the normal parent closer to you, one after the other. Notice that when the Deaf parent contributes a gene for normal hearing (blue chip), the offspring will have normal hearing. This is true for pairings of each gene from the normal-hearing parent. For these two possible gene pairings, the offspring would have normal hearing.

In total, there were four possible gene pairings for the offspring. Of these, two were predicted to produce deafness and two were predicted to result in normal hearing. In this illustration of autosomal dominant deafness, the odds are that 50%, or one half, of the offspring from these two parents will be Deaf.

Now, remove one of the blue chips and replace it with a white one. Form two pairs of chips in front of you, each having one white and one blue chip. In this case, the white chip represents the gene for deafness again, but it is recessive. The gene for normal hearing (blue chip) is dominant. There will again be four possible pairings of the chips in the offspring, one from each parent. Examine the various combinations of genes by first sliding one chip closer to you from the parent on the left. Examine two possible pairings for each gene from the parent on the right. Now repeat this process by sliding the other chip from the parent on the left closer to you. When you have finished, you should have observed the following four pairs of chips for the offspring (blue-white, blue-blue, white-blue, and white-white). In this case of autosomal recessive deafness, only one of the possible combinations would produce a Deaf offspring (white-white). The probability of a Deaf child is one in four, or 25%. Two of the three normal-hearing offspring, however, will carry a gene for deafness (blue-white chip pairs). These offspring are referred to as "carriers" of the trait.

It is sometimes difficult to understand that the Mendelian laws of hearing are only probabilities. In the case of autosomal recessive deafness, for example, one might think that if the parents had four offspring, then they would have one Deaf child. That is only the probability. They could very well have four normal-hearing children or four Deaf children. To see how this occurs, place one blue and one white chip in each of the two paper cups. Shake up the left cup and draw a chip. Repeat the process with the right cup. Examine the two chips (genes) selected, one from each cup (parent). Record the outcome (Deaf or normal hearing) and replace chips in the cups. Do this 20 times, representing five families of four offspring each. When you're finished, you will likely find some families of four that had two, three, or four Deaf offspring. If you did this an infinite number of times, however, 25% of the offspring would be Deaf, as predicted by Mendelian laws for autosomal recessive deafness.

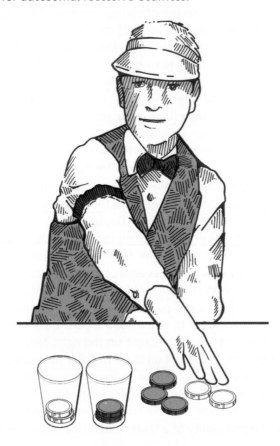

receive their Y chromosomes from their fathers; their X chromosomes are inherited from their mothers. Daughters, on the other hand, receive one X chromosome from their fathers and the other from their mothers. Approximately 2% to 3% of deafness occurs as a result of X-linked inheritance. Examples of autosomal dominant, recessive, and sex-linked syndromic forms of hereditary deafness are listed in Table 4.1.

Advances in Hereditary Deafness

The progress made in genetic research during the past 20 years has been truly remarkable and, subsequently, is continually changing our current understanding of hereditary deafness. Through gene mapping (identifying the chromosomal location of the gene) and localization (isolating the gene responsible for a disorder), it is now possible to identify genes responsible for deafness. Currently, the chromosomal locations of approximately 35 genes for nonsyndromic deafness have been mapped. For example, in 1997, a specific gene (GJB2 or Connexin 26) was identified that appears to be the cause of sensorineural hearing loss in many individuals. By testing for this gene alone, it is possible to identify the cause of deafness in as many as 40% of individuals in whom the cause of deafness was previously unknown. Identifying the genes that cause hearing loss may ultimately lead to therapeutic or preventive intervention in persons who exhibit genetic hearing impairment. Moreover, the possibility of genetic screening to determine the diagnosis after identification of hearing loss is now a topic of widespread discussion. Genetic screening may have important benefits for both the child and the child's parents. Genetic testing and counseling can assist families in learning more about the cause of hearing loss to determine the probability of recurring risks and to accept a diagnosis of deafness.

Site of Lesion

Also important in the classification of an auditory disorder is the location of the lesion. Disorders of the outer or middle ear cause a type of hearing loss, known as *conductive* hearing loss (Chapter 5), that is frequently amenable to medical treatment. If damage occurs to the nerve endings or to the hair cells in the inner ear, the hearing loss is termed *sensorineural* (Chapter 5). Hearing losses resulting from damage to the auditory nerve after it leaves the cochlea are sometimes designated neural or *retrocochlear*. When damage occurs to the nerve pathways within the auditory central nervous system (Chapter 3), the resulting condition is often known as *central* auditory impairment. So, the label used to describe the type of hearing loss—conductive, sensorineural, retrocochlear, or central—identifies the general location in the communication chain where the break or lesion occurs.

One other variable that can be used in the classification of auditory disorders, but that does not require detailed explanation here, is time of onset. Typically, the hearing loss is described, in part, with consideration of when the impairment was thought to occur (i.e., before delivery or after birth; before language development or after). Time of onset will be discussed in more detail later in this chapter.

Outer ear and middle ear disorders do not pose as serious a threat to the development and use of the communication chain as disorders located in the inner ear. This is basically because most outer ear and middle ear disorders are medically treatable once diagnosed, and do not result in long-term loss of input to the higher centers of the communication chain. Moreover, the hearing impairments associated with middle-ear problems, in general, tend to be less severe, often mild in degree; this, together with the loss typically being temporary, poses a less serious threat to the communication chain. As a result, the disorders reviewed in this chapter primarily involve the cochlea and result in permanent sensorineural hearing loss of varying degrees. One clear exception to this, however, involves a middle ear disorder known as chronic **otitis media.** This is a very prevalent disorder among young children and, despite diagnosis and medical treatment, can be a persistent hearing problem (hence the name "chronic" otitis media). As a result, this chapter first describes this middle ear disease and then moves on to those disorders resulting in sensorineural hearing loss.

THE PROBLEM OF OTITIS MEDIA

An important middle ear disorder frequently seen by the clinician is otitis media, one of the most common diseases in childhood. Otitis media refers to inflammation of the middle ear cavity. It is considered an important economic and health problem because of its prevalence, the cost of its treatment, the potential for secondary medical complications, and the possibility of long-term nonmedical consequences. The clinician must be familiar with this middle ear disorder and have a grasp of such important topics as the classification of otitis media, its natural history and epidemiology, its cause, its management, and its potential complications.

Classification of Otitis Media

Otitis media is often classified on the basis of the temporal sequence of the disease. In other words, the disease is categorized according to the duration of the disease process. For example, acute otitis media typically will run its full course within a 3-week period. The disease begins with a rapid onset, persists for a week to 10 days, and then resolves rapidly. Some of the more common symptoms associated with acute otitis media include a bulging, reddened tympanic membrane, pain, and upper respiratory infection. If the disease has a slow onset and persists for 3 months or more, it is referred to as chronic otitis media. Symptoms associated with chronic otitis media may include a large central perforation in the eardrum and discharge of fluid through the perforation. Subacute otitis media refers to a disease that has persisted beyond the acute stage but has not yet become chronic.

Otitis media is also classified according to the type of fluid that is observed by the physician in the middle ear cavity. If the fluid is purulent or suppurative, like the fluid found most often in acute otitis media, it will contain white blood cells, some cellular debris, and many bacteria. Acute otitis media is sometimes referred to as acute suppurative otitis media or acute purulent otitis media. A fluid that is free of cellular debris and bacteria is described as serous, and the term serous otitis media is used to describe this condition. Sometimes the fluid is mucoid because it has been secreted from the mucosal lining of the middle ear. This fluid is thick in substance and contains white blood cells, few bacteria, and some cellular debris. When mucoid fluid is present, the disease may be referred to as mucoid otitis media, or secretory otitis media. Table 4.2 summarizes the most commonly employed descriptions of otitis media and their associated synonyms. In addition, Figure 4.2 illustrates a normal tympanic membrane along with several pathologic conditions including serous otitis media, otitis media with bubbles in the fluid, and acute otitis media.

Natural History and Epidemiology of Otitis Media

To understand fully the nature of otitis media, one must appreciate the natural history and epidemiology of the disease. Natural history and epidemiology are terms used to denote the study of the relationships of various factors that determine the natural frequency and distribution of a disease. It has already been stated that otitis media with effusion is one of the most prevalent diseases in childhood (Vignette 4.2). Depending on the study reviewed, 76% to 95% of all

TABLE 4.2 **Clinical Classification of Otitis Media and Commonly Used Synonyms**

Classification	Synonyms
Otitis media without effusion	Myringitis
Acute otitis media	Suppurative OM, purulent OM, bacterial OM
Otitis media with effusion	Secretory OM, nonsuppurative OM, Serous OM, mucoid OM Suppurative OM, purulent OM

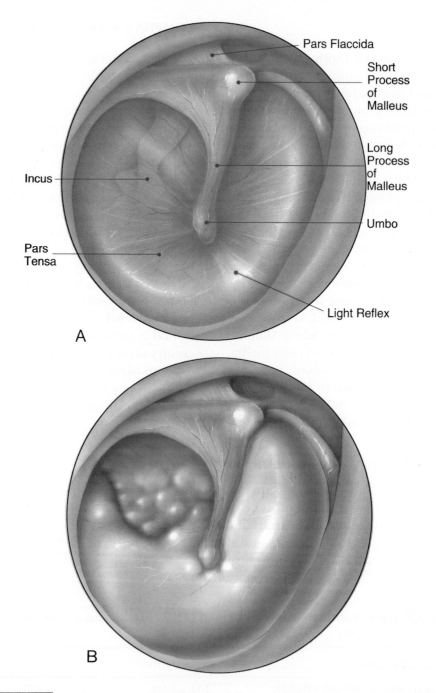

FIGURE 4.2 Normal tympanic membrane (*A*) and three pathologic conditions: serous otitis media (*B*), serous otitis media with air bubbles (*C*), and acute otitis media (*D*). (From English GM. *Otolaryngology*. Hagerstown, MD: Harper & Row; 1976, with permission.)

(Continued)

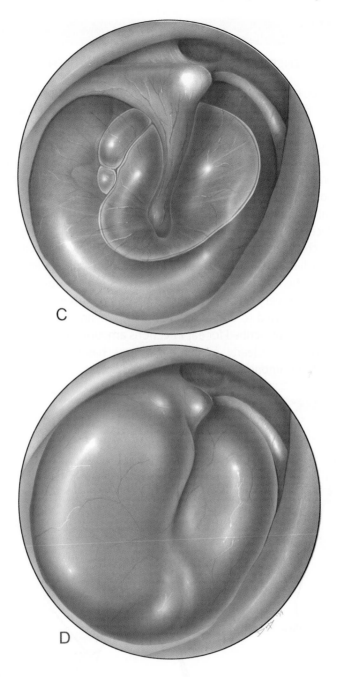

FIGURE 4.2 Continued

VIGNETTE 4.2   FURTHER DISCUSSION

PREVALENCE OF MIDDLE EAR DISEASE IN CHILDREN

The prevalence of middle ear disease has reached epidemic proportions. For children below the age of 6 years, otitis media is the most common reason for a doctor visit. It is estimated that one visit in three that is made for illness results in the diagnosis of middle ear disease. According to the National Center for Health Statistics, ear infection diagnoses increased 150% between 1975 and 1990. Moreover, in 1975, there were 10 million doctor visits for earaches; by 1990, there were 24.5 million visits, costing more than $1 billion annually. Nine out of every 10 children will have at least one ear infection; most will have at least one acute ear infection by age 3, and more than one third of all children will have three acute infections. Why is the prevalence of ear infections increasing? Many authorities believe that childcare is a significant factor. Children in daycare facilities experience a much higher prevalence of upper respiratory infections and, subsequently, ear infections.

The extent of the management for ear infections is also substantial. For example, the most common surgery on children is myringotomy with insertion tubes (Figs. 4.4 and 4.5), a procedure used to drain fluid and restore hearing. In addition, the cost of antibiotics commonly prescribed for ear infections amounts to several billion dollars in annual worldwide sales. Clearly, middle ear disease has become one of the major health care problems among children in the United States.

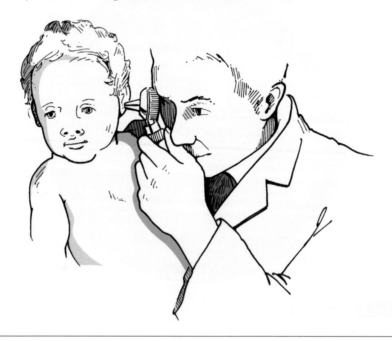

children have at least one episode of otitis media by 6 years of age. In addition, the prevalence of the disease peaks during the early years of life. The prevalence of otitis media is typically greatest during the first 2 years of life and then decreases with increasing age. Importantly, there appears to be a relationship between the age of onset and the probability of repeated episodes. Children who appear to be prone to middle ear disease and experience five to six bouts within the first several years of life have usually experienced their first episode of the disease during the first 18 months of life. Seldom does a child become otitis-prone if the first episode occurred after 18 months of age.

Otitis media varies slightly with sex, with more cases seen in males than in females. There is seasonal variation in otitis media, with higher occurrence during winter and spring. Some groups are more at risk for middle ear disease than others. Some of the groups considered more at risk for otitis media are children with cleft palate and other craniofacial disorders, those with Down syndrome, and those with learning disabilities. Children who reside in the inner city and children who attend daycare centers are also prone to suffer from middle ear disease, as are Native Americans.

Cause of Otitis Media

It is commonly believed that otitis media develops because of eustachian tube obstruction. As mentioned in Chapter 3, the eustachian tube is important to a healthy middle ear because it provides for pressure equalization and fluid drainage. If the pressure-equalization system is obstructed, a negative pressure can develop in the middle ear cavity. The negative pressure literally sucks the fluid from the membranous lining of the middle ear canal. The fluid that has accumulated from the mucosal lining of the middle ear has no place to escape because the eustachian tube is blocked. Vignette 4.3 shows a representation of this general process. A number of factors may produce eustachian tube obstruction, including large adenoid tissue in the nasopharyngeal area and inflammation of the mucous lining of the tube. It is also important to note that the muscular opening function of the eustachian tube is poor in children with otitis media and in children with histories of middle ear disease. In fact, in general, the muscle responsible for opening and closing the tube (tensor veli palatini) is less efficient among young infants and children. Moreover, the position of the eustachian tube in children lies at an angle of only 10 degrees in relation to the horizontal plane, whereas in adults this angle is 45 degrees (Fig. 4.3). Further, the tube is much shorter in infants. Because of the angle and shortness of the tube in children, fluid is able to reach the middle ear from the nasopharyngeal area with greater ease and has greater difficulty escaping from the middle ear cleft.

VIGNETTE 4.3   FURTHER DISCUSSION

DEVELOPMENT OF ACUTE OTITIS MEDIA

The figures that accompany this vignette illustrate the general pattern of events that can occur in acute otitis media. Panel A shows the landmarks of a normal middle ear system. Note the translucency and concavity of the tympanic membrane. Note also the appearance of the eustachian tube, especially at the opening in the nasopharyngeal area. Panel B shows that the pharyngeal end of the eustachian tube has been

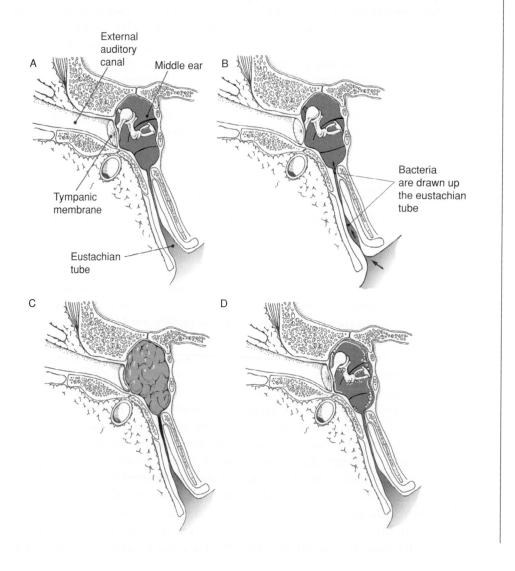

closed off by swelling because of pharyngeal infection or possibly an allergy. More specifically, the upper respiratory infection produces a congestion of the mucosa in the nasopharyngeal area, the eustachian tube, and the middle ear. The congestion of the mucosa of the tube produces an obstruction that prevents ventilation of the middle ear space. Also, the tympanic membrane is retracted inward because of negative pressure caused by absorption from the middle ear. Finally, bacteria from the oral pharyngeal area are drawn up the eustachian tube to the middle ear space. Panel C illustrates a full-blown condition of acute otitis media. Fluid secretions from the goblet cells of the mucosal lining of the middle ear are now trapped and have no way to leave the middle ear cavity. The bacteria drawn from the eustachian tube proliferate in the secretions, forming viscous pus. Observe also that the tympanic membrane is no longer retracted but is bulging.

Panel D shows a condition that may well result after antimicrobial treatment. The bacteria have been killed by the antibiotics, and a thin or mucoid-type fluid remains. Other possible outcomes after medical treatment might be the return to a completely normal middle ear, as in A, or a condition like the one shown in B.

The onset of otitis media with effusion, although asymptomatic, would follow a similar pattern of events. Recurrent episodes of acute otitis media or middle ear disease with effusion are probably a result of abnormal anatomy or physiology of the eustachian tube.

Hearing loss is considered the most common complication of otitis media. Although the type of the loss is usually conductive because the problem is located in the middle ear, sensorineural or inner ear involvement can also occur, especially in long-standing cases of otitis media. The hearing loss is usually flat, affecting all frequencies equally, and is mild in degree, usually around a 25-dB hearing loss for mid-frequency pure tones (500 to 2,000 Hz). The degree of hearing loss in individual cases, though, can range from normal sensitivity to hearing losses as great as 50 dB. In general, the prevalence rate for hearing loss associated with otitis media depends on the criteria used to define hearing loss. Unfortunately, prevalence data are difficult to determine because of the lack of well-controlled studies in this area.

Another complication that may result from longstanding middle ear disease with effusion is deficiency in psychoeducational and/or communicative skills. It is widely suspected that otitis-prone children are more susceptible to delays in speech, language, and cognitive development, and in education. The research findings in this area, however, are inconclusive, and a cause-effect

INFANT EAR

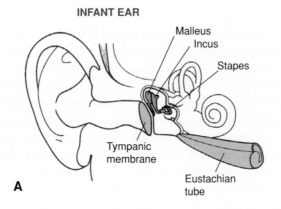

A

ADULT EAR

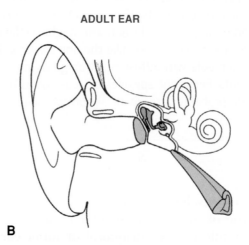

B

FIGURE 4.3   Anatomic illustration of the eustachian tube in an infant ear (A) compared with that of the adult ear (B). Note that the tube of an infant lies more on a horizontal plane.

relationship cannot be assumed at the present time. Clearly, given our understanding of the development of the communication chain, if chronic otitis media resulted in a mild or mild-to-moderate hearing loss of 25 to 50 dB that developed at an early age (<18 months) and the hearing loss persisted for many months, a negative effect on the development of communication skills *could* occur. As a result, the key is the identification and treatment of otitis media early in the development of the disease.

Management of Otitis Media

A common means of treating acute otitis media is the routine administration of antimicrobial agents. These antibiotics are designed to combat the various pathogens thought to exist within the middle ear fluid. Pharmaceutical agents, such as ampicillin, amoxicillin, erythromycin, and amoxicillin/clavulanic (Augmentin), are frequently administered in the management of acute otitis media. Unfortunately, the overall effectiveness of antibiotic therapy in the treatment of ear disease has not been clearly established. Even when appropriate antimicrobial agents have been prescribed and the fluid is sterilized, the effusion may persist for 2 weeks to 3 months. Also, antibiotic medications can produce adverse side effects such as diarrhea, nausea, vomiting, and skin rash. Finally, antihistamines and decongestants have also been used in the treatment of middle ear disease; however, this form of treatment has been shown to be ineffective.

A common surgical approach to the management of both suppurative and nonsuppurative otitis media is a myringotomy. Myringotomy is a surgical procedure that involves making an incision in one of the inferior quadrants of the tympanic membrane, as shown in Figure 4.4. In the acute forms of the

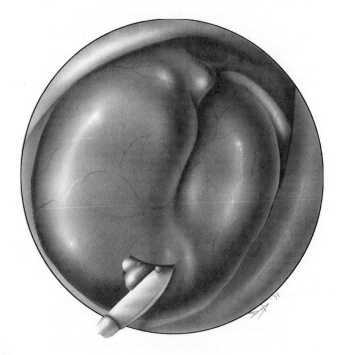

FIGURE 4.4 Myringotomy. Note the bulging appearance of the tympanic membrane. (From English GM. *Otolaryngology*. Hagerstown, MD: Harper & Row; 1976.)

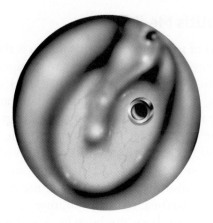

FIGURE 4.5 Ventilating tube or grommet.

disease, a myringotomy is performed when there is severe pain or toxicity, high fever, failure to respond to antimicrobial therapy, or some serious secondary medical complication. In secretory otitis media, a myringotomy is more commonly performed, usually to remove fluid and restore hearing sensitivity. This surgical procedure is performed in cases where the disease has persisted for at least 3 months. The eardrum incision can heal quickly, however, and the fluid reappears. To avoid this possibility and to ensure sustained middle ear aeration, ventilating tubes or grommets are often inserted into the eardrum (Fig. 4.5).

Tonsillectomy and adenoidectomy are also considered as a management approach to otitis media. Although tonsillectomy does not seem to be an effective treatment protocol, adenoidectomy is a common surgical procedure for the management of bilateral otitis media in children 4 years of age or older. In general, this approach is undertaken when a patient does not respond to medical therapy, large adenoids are present, and there is no evidence of nasal allergy. Under these conditions, it is assumed that the eustachian tube blockage causing the middle ear disease is a result of enlarged adenoids. The adenoids are removed to free the eustachian tube from the blockage.

A more radical surgical approach is required if chronic disease permanently impairs basic structures within the middle ear. When alteration of the middle ear structures is required, a surgical technique known as tympanoplasty is performed. Tympanoplasty may simply involve repair of a chronically perforated eardrum or may also involve reconstruction of ossicles that have been eroded away by the longstanding disease.

COCHLEAR AND RETROCOCHLEAR PATHOLOGY

Millions of Americans have sensorineural hearing loss as a consequence of cochlear pathology. For children, conductive hearing loss produced by middle ear pathology, as reviewed earlier in this chapter, is probably the most common type of hearing loss. For adults, however, sensorineural hearing loss resulting from underlying cochlear pathology is probably the most common type of hearing impairment. Recall from the previous sections of this chapter that conductive hearing loss is usually medically treatable, either through surgery, medication, or a combination of the two. With sensorineural hearing loss, however, this is usually not the case. The hearing loss is typically permanent. For those individuals with significant sensorineural hearing loss, the usual course of action is to seek assistance from amplification, often a personal wearable hearing aid. Hearing aids and other types of amplification for the hearing impaired are described in detail in Chapter 7.

The description of the hearing loss produced by cochlear pathology as "sensorineural" seems particularly appropriate. The presence of a sensorineural hearing loss does not tell us the exact location of the pathology along the auditory pathway (Chapter 5); it only eliminates the outer and middle ears as possibilities. The pathology could be affecting the sensory receptors within the cochlea, or the neural pathways leading from the cochlea to higher centers of the auditory system, or both the sensory and neural structures. In this context, then, "sensorineural" hearing loss is a very appropriate label.

The term sensorineural hearing loss is also an appropriate label for the hearing loss resulting from cochlear pathology for another reason. In cochlear pathology, the sensory receptors within the cochlea are destroyed. Exactly how this occurs depends on the specific etiology. Research suggests that the sensory destruction quickly becomes sensorineural damage. Once the inner hair cells within the organ of Corti are destroyed, a phenomenon known as retrograde degeneration occurs. *Retrograde degeneration* refers to the destruction of connecting anatomic structures located more central to the structure that was destroyed. Destruction of the inner hair cells within the organ of Corti results in the eventual degeneration of the first-order afferent nerve fibers communicating with the damaged hair cells. Most patients with profound sensorineural hearing loss caused by cochlear pathology, therefore, most likely have underlying damage to both the sensory (cochlea) and neural (nerve fibers) portions of the peripheral auditory system.

When a sensorineural hearing loss is observed, how do the audiologist and physician determine whether it is because of cochlear pathology or a problem further up the ascending neural pathways (called **retrocochlear pathology**)?

Several steps are involved in establishing the diagnosis (Chapter 5). The case history taken by the audiologist or physician can provide some important clues as to the location of the problem. The presence of other (frequently nonauditory) complaints, such as dizziness, loss of balance, and ringing in the ears (tinnitus), can aid the physician in establishing the diagnosis. A particular pattern of results from the basic audiology test battery may alert the physician to a probable underlying cause. Finally, special tests can be performed on the patient at the physician's request. These tests may be auditory, in which case they will be performed by an audiologist, or they may be nonauditory. An example of a nonauditory special test is electronystagmography, which tests the vestibular system and may also be performed by an audiologist. Another nonauditory test, one not performed by the audiologist, might involve some form of tomography. Tomography provides a visual image of the brain and brainstem structures. Computed tomography (CT) scans are increasingly commonplace. The most definitive auditory special test involves the measurement of the auditory brainstem response (ABR). This test may also be administered by an audiologist. (The ABR was described briefly in Chapter 3.)

Discussion of the special tests, auditory and nonauditory, that aid the physician in establishing the diagnosis is beyond the scope of this book. Suffice it to say that such tests exist and that the audiologist is frequently asked to perform them. Many types of cochlear and retrocochlear pathology, however, do produce distinct patterns of hearing loss and can result in breaks in the communication chain. The remainder of this chapter describes several of these more common pathologies.

Cochlear Pathology

Before describing some specific causes of cochlear pathology, some general characteristics shared by most patients with cochlear pathology are noteworthy. First, for the most part, studies of human cadavers have revealed a close correspondence between the location of the damage along the length of the cochlea and the resulting audiometric configuration. For example, if postmortem anatomic studies of a patient's ear reveal damage in the basal high-frequency portion of the cochlea, then a recent audiogram obtained before death would most likely indicate the presence of a high-frequency sensorineural hearing loss. Although there are exceptions, it is generally the case in cochlear pathology that the pattern of hearing loss or audiometric configuration provides at least a gross indication of the regions of the cochlea that were damaged by the pathology. A high-frequency sensorineural hearing loss reflects damage to the basal portion of the cochlea, a low-frequency sensorineural hearing loss suggests damage to the apical region of the cochlea, and a broad hearing loss extending from low to high frequencies reflects an underlying lesion along the entire length of the cochlea. This follows directly from the mapping of sound frequency to place of maximum mechanical activity in the cochlea, or tonotopic organization, noted previously in Chapter 3.

In sensorineural hearing loss caused by cochlear pathology, there is a close correspondence between the frequencies that demonstrate hearing loss and the region along the length of the cochlea that is damaged. There is a less certain correspondence, however, between the degree of hearing loss at a particular frequency and the degree of damage at the corresponding location in the cochlea. One popular conception is that mild or moderate degrees of sensorineural hearing loss result from destruction of the outer hair cells, whereas more severe hearing loss reflects damage to both the outer and inner hair cells of the cochlea.

There are also several perceptual consequences of sensorineural hearing loss caused by cochlear pathology. Except for those with profound impairments, patients with cochlear pathology most commonly complain that they can hear speech, but cannot understand it. This may be especially true when listening against a background of noise. The reason for this common complaint in many individuals with cochlear pathology is that it is often the basal portion of the cochlea that is most severely damaged in cochlear pathology. This results in a hearing loss for high-frequency sounds. Many important consonant sounds, such as "s", "t," and "f", are low-intensity, high-frequency speech sounds. An individual who has trouble hearing high-frequency sounds will often not be able to hear these speech sounds. They will, however, be able to hear many other speech sounds, such as vowels, because these sounds have most of their energy in the lower frequencies where hearing is normal or close to normal in these individuals. When this individual is presented with a series of words such as "white, wife, wipe, wise," what is perceived may be something like "why, why, why, why" because the high-frequency consonants are too soft to be heard. As a result, the individual can tell that someone is speaking, but cannot understand what is said. This, of course, can cause a breakdown in communication between the talker and the listener.

Hearing Loss Demonstration

The patient with cochlear pathology also frequently experiences a phenomenon known as loudness recruitment. The hearing loss makes low-intensity sounds inaudible. Moderate-intensity sounds that are comfortably loud to a normal-hearing person may be barely audible to the person with cochlear pathology. At high intensities, however, the loudness of the sound is the same for both a normal ear and one with cochlear pathology. Let us assume, for example, that a pure tone at 2,000 Hz having a level of 110 dB SPL is uncomfortably loud for both a normal listener and a person with cochlear pathology. The person with cochlear pathology, however, has a hearing threshold at 2,000 Hz of 60 dB SPL, whereas the normal listener's threshold is 10 dB SPL. Thus, for the normal listener, the intensity of the tone has to be increased 100 dB to increase the loudness of the tone from "just audible" (threshold) to "uncomfortable." For the person with cochlear pathology, however, an increase in intensity of only 50 dB is needed to cover the same range of loudness (from "just audible" to "uncomfortable"). Loudness increases more rapidly in the ear with cochlear pathology than in the normal ear. This is known as loudness recruitment.

The presence of loudness recruitment makes it more difficult to fit a hearing aid on a person with cochlear pathology. Low-level sounds need to be amplified to be made audible to the hearing-impaired person. High-intensity sounds, however, cannot be amplified by the same amount or the hearing aid will produce sounds that are uncomfortably loud to the wearer. Possible solutions to this dilemma when fitting the patient with a hearing aid are described in more detail in Chapter 7.

Finally, the patient with cochlear hearing loss may have accompanying speech abnormalities. As noted previously, the auditory system of the talker or sender is also used to monitor the quality of the acoustic speech sounds produced by the talker. Depending on the severity, configuration, and age of onset of the hearing loss, the talker's speech may be misarticulated. In addition, if the cochlear pathology produces sensorineural hearing loss in the low and intermediate frequencies, the patient will typically use speech levels that are inappropriately loud, especially while talking without wearing a hearing aid. This is because the feedback that a speaker normally receives is not available to assist in regulating the voice level.

Now that we have reviewed some features shared by most individuals with cochlear pathology, the remainder of this section will examine several types of pathology. The pathologies described here are by no means an exhaustive compilation. In keeping with the general mission of this book, the pathologies described were selected either because of their common occurrence in the general population or among children or because of their potential for severe negative impact on the communication chain.

Viral and Bacterial Diseases

Severe viral and bacterial infections can result in varying degrees and patterns of sensorineural hearing loss. Infectious disease can be transmitted to the child by the mother in utero, a condition referred to as prenatal, congenital, or sometimes perinatal disease. These terms carry slightly different meanings, yet are often used synonymously. The term *prenatal* refers to something that occurs to the fetus before birth. *Congenital* also implies before birth, but usually before the 28th week of gestation. *Perinatal* pertains to a condition that occurs in the

TABLE 4.3	(S)TORCH Complex of High-Risk Prenatal Infections
S	Syphilis
T	Toxoplasmosis
O	Other
R	Rubella
C	Cytomegalovirus
H	Herpes simplex virus

period shortly before or after birth (from 8 weeks before birth to 4 weeks after). A disease can also be acquired later in life; this is usually referred to as a *postnatal* condition. The following discussion reviews some of the more common prenatal and postnatal infectious diseases known to cause hearing loss.

Prenatal Diseases   Many of the prenatal diseases are categorized as part of the TORCH complex, an acronym used to identify the major infections that may be contracted in utero (*t*oxoplasmosis, *o*ther, *r*ubella, *c*ytomegalovirus, and *her*pes simplex virus). Some have used the mnemonic (S)TORCH, where S stands for syphilis. Any disease of the (S)TORCH complex is considered a high-risk factor for hearing loss, and therefore it is important for the audiologist to have some general knowledge of these infectious conditions. Table 4.3 lists the (S)TORCH diseases.

Postnatal Infections   Several postnatal infections produce sensorineural hearing loss. The cochlear damage produced by these viral or bacterial infections appears to result from the infecting agent entering the inner ear through the blood supply and nerve fibers. The following is a brief review of those diseases that would be encountered most frequently.

Hearing loss is the most common consequence of acute meningitis. Although the pathways used by the organisms to reach the inner ear are not altogether clear, several routes have been suggested. These include the bloodstream, the auditory nerve, and the fluid supply of the inner ear and the middle ear. The prevalence of severe-to-profound sensorineural hearing loss among patients with this disorder is approximately 10%. Another 16% will exhibit transient conductive hearing loss. Interestingly, some patients with sensorineural hearing loss will exhibit partial recovery, although such a finding is rare.

Mumps is recognized as one of the more common causes of sensorineural hearing loss that affects just one ear (unilateral hearing loss). The hearing loss is usually sudden and can vary from mild high-frequency impairment to profound loss. Both children and adults are affected. Because it is not uncommon for this disease to be subclinical, children with hearing loss resulting from mumps are not usually identified until they first attend school.

Measles is another cause of sensorineural hearing loss. Hearing loss affects 6% to 10% of measles patients. A typical pattern of hearing loss shows a severe to profound hearing loss for high frequencies and in both ears.

Ototoxic Drugs

A negative side effect of some antibiotic drugs is the production of severe high-frequency sensorineural hearing loss. A group of antibiotics known as aminoglycosides are particularly hazardous. This group, also commonly referred to as the "mycin" drugs, includes streptomycin, neomycin, kanamycin, and gentamicin. A variety of factors can determine whether hearing loss is produced in a specific patient. These factors include the drug dosage, the susceptibility of the patient, and the simultaneous or previous use of other ototoxic agents.

Ototoxic antibiotics reach the inner ear through the bloodstream. The resulting damage is greater in the base of the cochlea, and outer hair cells are typically the primary targets, with only limited damage appearing in other cochlear structures. This results in a pattern of hearing loss that is moderate to severe in the high frequencies of both ears.

Some ototoxic drugs cause a temporary or reversible hearing loss. Perhaps the most common such substance is aspirin. When taken in large amounts, aspirin can produce a mild to moderate temporary sensorineural hearing loss.

Noise-Induced Hearing Loss

Exposure to intense sounds can result in temporary or permanent hearing loss. Whether or not a hearing loss actually results from exposure to the intense sound depends on several factors. These factors include the acoustic characteristics of the sound such as its intensity, duration, and frequency content (amplitude spectrum), the length of the exposure, and the susceptibility of the individual.

When the intense sound is a broadband noise, such as might be found in industrial settings, a characteristic pattern of hearing loss emerges after the exposure. This pattern is frequently referred to as a "4k notch" and reflects the sharp loss of hearing that is maximized at 4 kHz. More detailed measurements of the hearing loss produced by exposure to broadband noise reveal that the sharp drop in hearing threshold is as likely to appear at 3 or 6 kHz as at 4 kHz. Because 3 and 6 kHz are not routinely included in audiometric testing

(Chapter 5), however, the notch is less frequently observed at these two frequencies. This same "4k notch" configuration is observed both in temporary hearing loss after brief exposures to broadband noise and in permanent hearing loss after prolonged exposure to such noise.

Many theories attempt to explain why the region around 4 kHz seems to be more susceptible to the damaging effects of broadband noise. One theory is that, although the noise itself may be broadband, with roughly equal amplitude at all frequencies, the outer ear and ear canal resonances (Chapter 3) have amplified the noise in the 2 to 4 kHz region by the time the noise reaches the inner ear. Thus, this region shows the greatest hearing loss. Other theories suggest that the region of the cochlea associated with 4 kHz is more vulnerable to damage because of differences in cochlear mechanics, cochlear metabolism, or cochlear blood supply. Whatever the underlying mechanism, damage is greatest in that region of the cochlea associated with 3 to 6 kHz. The damage again seems to be more marked in the outer hair cells, although this can vary with the acoustic characteristics of the noise.

Given the permanent nature of the resulting noise-induced hearing loss, it is crucial to prevent its occurrence. Hearing conservation programs have been developed by employers to protect the hearing of their employees. At least part of the employer's motivation is the avoidance of hefty fines for noncompliance with federal standards regarding industrial noise levels. Basically, the primary components of an industrial hearing conservation program include surveys of noise levels and durations to which employees are exposed, regular (at least annual) monitoring of hearing thresholds for all employees, and the provision of hearing protection devices, such as earmuffs and earplugs. A key component of such hearing conservation programs also involves the education of employees regarding the risk of permanent hearing loss from noise exposure and instruction in the effective use of hearing protection devices.

The world in which we live, however, is increasingly noisy. Exposure to high noise levels is not confined to work environments. Many recreational sources of noise exist today, and the risk of hearing loss from prolonged exposure to high sound levels is the same whether it involves a 110-dB SPL machine-generated noise or an exposure to 110-dB SPL from loudspeakers at a rock concert (Vignette 4.4). The biggest difference in these two cases, however, is that an employee might be exposed to the high-level machine-generated noise on a daily basis for many years, whereas the audience member at a rock concert will most likely be exposed to this same high noise level much less frequently. Of course, if one considers the rock musician, including practices and performances, the differences in exposure duration and the subsequent risk of hearing loss might be minimal. Musicians, however, are no

VIGNETTE 4.4 FURTHER DISCUSSION

RECREATIONAL SOURCES OF NOISE

We live in a noise-filled society in which many recreational activities make use of devices or equipment that generate high levels of sound. In many cases, those making

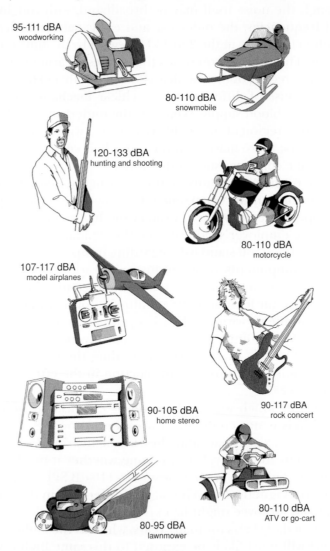

95-111 dBA
woodworking

80-110 dBA
snowmobile

120-133 dBA
hunting and shooting

80-110 dBA
motorcycle

107-117 dBA
model airplanes

90-117 dBA
rock concert

90-105 dBA
home stereo

80-110 dBA
ATV or go-cart

80-95 dBA
lawnmower

(Adapted from Clark WW, Bohne BA. The effects of noise on hearing and the ear. *Med Times*. 1984;122:17–22.)

use of these devices may not consider the sound to be "noise," but it is nonetheless high-intensity sound. The figure shows several recreational sources of noise In each case, the range of maximum sound levels in dBA* reported in various studies is shown.

*Instruments used to measure noise have three weighting networks (A, B, and C) that are designed to respond differently to noise frequencies. The A network weighs (filters) the low frequencies and approximates the response characteristics of the human ear. The B network also filters the low frequencies, but not as much as the A network does. The C scale provides a fairly flat response. The federal government recommends the A network for measuring noise levels.

longer the only ones who could be exposed to high levels of music for long periods of time. For example, contemporary MP3 audio players allow long, uninterrupted periods of music listening; the small size, long battery life, and expansive memory capabilities of these devices enable uninterrupted playback of hundreds of songs. When combined with volume controls that enable outputs in the listener's ears of over 110 dB SPL, the potential risk to hearing from such devices has raised concerns among many hearing health-care professionals.

Presbycusis

After approximately 60 years of age, hearing sensitivity deteriorates progressively, especially in the high frequencies. The progression, known as **presbycusis,** is somewhat more rapid for men than for women. Figure 4.6 shows the progression of hearing loss in both men and women as a function of age. The more rapid decline of hearing with age in men may not reflect differences in aging per se, but may reflect their more frequent participation in noisy recreational activities such as hunting, snowmobiling, or operating power tools (e.g., lawn mowers, chain saws, and table saws).

The patterns of hearing loss associated with ototoxic antibiotics, noise-induced hearing loss, and presbycusis are all very similar. In all three cases, a bilateral high-frequency sensorineural hearing loss is usually observed. The underlying cochlear damage is also very similar: the basal high-frequency region of the cochlea is the main area of destruction and the outer hair cells are primarily affected. Accompanying retrograde destruction of first-order afferent nerve fibers may also be observed, as is usually the case in cochlear pathology.

Degenerative changes associated with aging have also been observed in the brainstem and cortical areas of the ascending auditory pathway in some cases. These central changes, when present, can seriously compound the

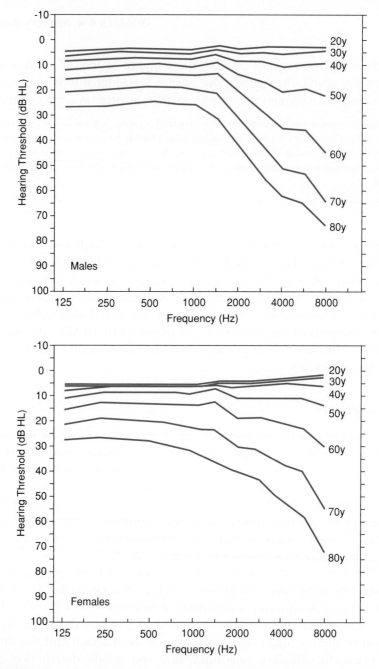

FIGURE 4.6 Hearing loss progression as a function of age in men (top) and women (bottom). Perfectly normal hearing is represented in these graphs by the horizontal line at 0 dB. (Adapted from Johansson MS, Arlinger SD. Hearing threshold levels for an otologically unscreened, non-occupationally noise-exposed population in Sweden. *Int J Audiol.* 2002;41:180–194, with permission

communicative impairment experienced by the elderly person with sensorineural hearing loss. Approximately 5% to 15% of elderly persons may have central auditory deficits affecting their ability to communicate. Aging can also have a negative impact on some aspects of cognitive function, including memory and attention. Some of these cognitive processes are important for effective communication. In that regard, older adults may experience a double or triple "whammy" with regard to impairments that have a negative impact on the communication chain. They not only are likely to have some amount of high-frequency hearing loss from inner ear damage, but may also have impairments in central auditory function, cognitive function, or both.

Retrocochlear Pathology

Retrocochlear pathology refers to damage to nerve fibers along the ascending auditory pathways from the internal auditory meatus to the cortex. Most often a tumor is involved, although not always, as in the case of multiple sclerosis or cerebral vascular attack (CVA or "stroke").

In many cases, the auditory manifestations of the retrocochlear pathology are subtle. Frequently, for example, no hearing loss is measured for pure tones. The possibility that a tumor along the auditory pathway will fail to produce measurable hearing loss for pure tones can be understood when one recalls the multiple paths by which information ascends through the brainstem within the auditory system (Chapter 3). Recall that after the first-order ascending neurons terminated in the cochlear nucleus, a variety of paths were available for the neurally transmitted information to ascend to the cortex. Thus, if the tumor is located central to the cochlear nucleus, the information required for the detection of a pure tone can easily bypass the affected pathway and progress to the cortex.

For the detection of a pure tone, many of the brainstem centers along the ascending auditory pathways probably serve simple relay functions and perform little processing of the signal. For more complex signals, such as speech, however, some preprocessing probably takes place in the brainstem before complete processing by the cortex. Still, in many brainstem and cortical disorders, speech perception appears normal in quiet listening conditions. This seems to be accomplished through the use of multiple cues available in the speech signal that assist in its recognition. Some of the cues processed by a brainstem or a cortical center can be eliminated from the total information reaching the cortex by the presence of a tumor without producing a misperception of the speech signal. The patient is simply using several of the remaining cues that are not affected by the presence of the tumor. If, however, the speech signal is degraded by filtering, adding noise, temporal interruption, and so forth, the cues of the speech signal become less redundant. Every cue in the speech signal is now needed for its correct recognition. Individuals with retrocochlear pathology in the brainstem or cortex typically perform poorly on speech-recognition tests involving the recognition of degraded speech signals.

Again, a detailed description of retrocochlear disorders and the tests developed for their detection is beyond the scope of this book. Many special speech-recognition tests making use of degraded speech have been developed for use with this population.

SUMMARY

The auditory system, marvelously complex and intricate, is nevertheless vulnerable to assault and damage from disease, trauma, genetic imperfection, extreme environmental conditions (i.e., noise), and aging. Many conditions affect both children and adults and can affect all levels of the auditory system, resulting in various types, degrees, and patterns of hearing loss. These problems, in turn, can have a negative impact on the development and function of the communication chain.

CHAPTER REVIEW QUESTIONS

1. If both parents have normal hearing but carry the same genes for recessive hereditary deafness, what is the likelihood that they will have a child with impaired hearing?

2. Why is otitis media much more common among young children than adults?

3. List the prenatal infections that comprise the (S)TORCH complex. If the mother develops any of these prenatal infections during her pregnancy, does that mean that she will give birth to a child with impaired hearing?

4. What are three common forms of cochlear pathology in adults, each of which results in an inability to hear low-intensity, high-frequency sounds? What is the impact of such a hearing loss on speech communication?

5. Several viral infections that are prevalent (or have been prevalent in the past) among children can lead to severe or profound loss of hearing. Describe two of these viral infections and the most likely pattern of hearing loss that would result. For each, what do believe would be the impact of the hearing loss on communication? Would the age at which the hearing loss developed matter? Why or why not?

6. What is meant by "retrocochlear" pathology?

REFERENCES AND SUGGESTED READINGS

Bess FH. *Hearing Impairment in Children*. Parkton, MD: York Press; 1988.

Carhart R. Clinical application of bone conduction audiometry. *Arch Otolaryngol.* 1950;51:798–807.

Eichwald J, Mahoney T. Apgar scores in the identification of sensorineural hearing loss. *J Am Acad Audiol.* 1993;4:133–138.

English GM. *Otolaryngology.* Hagerstown, MD: Harper & Row; 1976.

Fria TJ, Cantekin EI, Eichler JA. Hearing acuity of children with otitis media with effusion. *Arch Otolaryngol.* 1985;111:10–16.

Gerkin KP. The high risk register for deafness. *ASHA.* 1984;26:17–23.

Goodhill V. *Ear Diseases, Deafness, and Dizziness.* Hagerstown, MD: Harper & Row; 1979.

Jerger J, Jerger S. *Auditory Disorders.* Boston: Little Brown; 1981.

Johansson MS, Arlinger SD. Hearing threshold levels for an otologically unscreened, non-occupationally noise-exposed population in Sweden. *Int J Audiol.* 2002;41:180–194.

Joint Committee on Infant Hearing. Year 2007 statement: Principles and guidelines for early hearing detection and intervention programs. *Pediatrics.* 2007;120:898–921.

Katz J. *Handbook of Clinical Audiology.* 6th ed. Baltimore: Lippincott, Williams, and Wilkins, in press.

Kavanaugh J. *Otitis Media and Child Development.* Parkton, MD: York Press; 1986.

Lebo CP, Reddell RC. The presbycusis component in occupational hearing loss. *Laryngoscope.* 1972;82:1399–1409.

Newton VE. *Pediatric Audiological Medicine.* Philadelphia, PA: Whurr Publishers; 2002.

Northern JL. *Hearing Disorders.* 4th ed. Boston: Little Brown; 1991.

Parving A. Congenital hearing disability epidemiology and identification: A comparison between two health authority districts. *Int J Pediatr Otorhinolaryngol.* 1993;27:29–46.

Rodgers GK, Telischi FF: Ménière's disease in children. *Otolaryngol Clin North Am.* 1997;30:1101–1104.

Shambaugh GE, Glasscock ME. *Surgery of the Ear.* Philadelphia: WB Saunders; 1980.

Shuknecht HF. *Pathology of the Ear.* Cambridge: Harvard University Press; 1974.

Tekin M, Arnos KS, Pandya A. Advances in hereditary deafness. *Lancet.* 2001; 358:1082–1090.

CHAPTER

5

Audiologic Measurement

CHAPTER OBJECTIVES

- To understand how audiologists measure hearing loss for pure tones and speech;
- To be able to interpret the graphical presentation of test results on an audiogram;
- To understand how immittance measurements are performed by the audiologist and how this information is presented graphically; and
- To see how each test of the basic audiological test battery provides an important piece of the puzzle in diagnosing the hearing loss, as well as understanding its impact on communication.

KEY TERMS AND DEFINITIONS

- **Pure-tone audiometry:** The measurement of hearing thresholds for pure tones of various frequencies using standardized equipment and procedures.

- **Speech audiometry:** The measurement of speech recognition threshold in decibels, representing the lowest sound level at which speech can be heard 50% of the time, and measures of the ability to understand speech when it is many decibels above this threshold. The latter is a speech-recognition score reported as a percentage and represents the percentage of spoken words on standardized lists that were correctly perceived by the patient. When individual words are used to measure the speech-recognition score, which is most often the case clinically, the score is referred to as the "word recognition score."

- **Acoustic immittance measurements:** Clinical measurement of the impedance or admittance of the flow of sound energy through the middle ear. Typically includes measurement of a tympanogram and acoustic reflex thresholds.

In the preceding chapters, the importance of an intact auditory system, from the periphery to the cortex, for the communication chain was emphasized. This system is critical for the conversion of acoustical speech sounds generated by the talker to neural signals that can be interpreted by the brain of the listener. Impairments of the auditory system, as reviewed in Chapter 4, have the potential to disrupt or break the communication chain. Much of audiology is devoted to the detection of such impairments, their location within the auditory system, and the determination of their severity and impact on communication. This chapter reviews some of the methods and test techniques used in audiology to accomplish these tasks. Because most readers of this text are unlikely to become audiologists themselves, the approach taken here is to provide enough information so that the reader can become an "intelligent consumer" of audiological information. As a result, in this chapter we focus on the results that are obtained by the audiologist and their interpretation, more than details about how such measurements are performed.

The nature of auditory impairment depends on such factors as the severity of the hearing loss, the age at onset, the cause of the loss, and the location of the lesion within the auditory system. The hearing evaluation plays an important role in determining some of these factors. Audiometric measurement of auditory function can: (a) determine the degree of hearing loss; (b) estimate the location of the lesion within the auditory system that is producing the problem; (c) help establish the cause of the hearing problem; (d) estimate the extent of the handicap produced by the hearing loss; and (e) help to determine the client's habilitative or rehabilitative needs and the appropriate means of filling those needs. This chapter will focus on those tests used most commonly in the evaluation of auditory function. This battery of tests includes pure-tone audiometry, speech audiometry, and acoustic immittance measures.

CASE HISTORY

Before the audiologic evaluation begins, the audiologist obtains a history from the client. For adults, this history may be supplied by completing a printed form before the evaluation. The form contains pertinent identifying information for the client, such as home address and referral source. Questions regarding the nature of past and present hearing problems, including a family history of hearing loss or a history of exposure to noise, other medical problems, and prior use of amplification are also usually included. The written responses are then followed up during an interview between the audiologist and the client before any testing.

For children, the case history form is usually more comprehensive than the adult version. In addition to questions such as the ones mentioned for adults, detailed questions about the mother's pregnancy and the child's birth are included. The development of gross and fine motor skills and the development of speech and language are also probed. The medical history of the child is also reviewed in detail, with special emphasis on childhood diseases (e.g., measles, mumps, etc.) capable of producing a hearing loss. Vignette 5.1 provides examples of common questions included on a pediatric case-history form used by audiologists.

OTOSCOPY

Once the case history has been completed, the audiologist will typically examine the patient's ear canals and eardrums with a small handheld otoscope prior to proceeding to pure-tone audiometry. A skilled audiologist will often be able to considerably narrow the list of possible auditory disorders for a particular case on the basis of the initial case history and otoscopy. The audiologist inspects the ear canal for the presence of foreign objects, excessive ear wax, signs of inflammation or irritation, dried blood, among other things. The appearance of the eardrum is also examined closely, with special attention paid to the coloration of the eardrum, whether it is distended or bulging, the opacity of the eardrum, the visibility of fluid in the middle ear, and the presence of any scars, perforations, or tears in the eardrum. A readily visible hallmark of a healthy eardrum and middle ear is referred to the "cone of light" and results from the reflection of the otoscope's light by the malleus. The cone of light appears as a brighter strip or narrow wedge of light located in the lower front quadrant of the eardrum (typically, between the 4 and 6 o'clock positions if the eardrum is visualized as the face of a clock).

PURE-TONE AUDIOMETRY

Pure-tone audiometry is the basis of a hearing evaluation. With pure-tone audiometry, hearing thresholds are measured for pure tones at different test frequencies. Hearing threshold is typically defined as the lowest (softest) sound level needed for a person to detect the presence of a signal approximately 50% of the time. Threshold information at each frequency is then plotted on a graph known as an audiogram. Before examining the audiogram, however, we shall describe the equipment used to measure hearing.

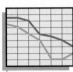

VIGNETTE 5.1   CLINICAL APPLICATIONS

EXAMPLE OF A PEDIATRIC CASE-HISTORY FORM USED IN AUDIOLOGY

Child over 4 years

Date: _____

Interviewer: _____

Name: _____   DOB: _____

Nature and Onset of Problem:
Chief complaint:

Duration:

Progression/consistency:

Communication difficulties:

Medical History:
Familial history of speech/hearing/other medical problems:

Unusual prenatal conditions:

Unusual postnatal conditions:

Serious childhood diseases/conditions:

Ear infections:

Speech-language Development:
Present speech-language behavior:

Past speech-language therapy:

Educational History:
Past educational concerns:

Present school progress:

Difficult academic subjects:

Preferential seating or extra academic help:

Special education services:

Child over 4 years

General Information: Date: _____

Name of child: _____   Age: _____

Informant: _____(relationship to child)

Who stays with the child during the day? _____

List other children in the family:

Name	Age	Grade	Speech and/or hearing problems?
_____	_____	_____	_____
_____	_____	_____	_____
_____	_____	_____	_____

Chief Concern:

_____

_____

_____

_____

How does s/he respond to various types of sounds such as speech, telephone ringing, music, whispered speech, television, etc.?_____

_____

_____

Are there any sounds that frighten him/her? _____

_____

Any unusual responses to sounds? _____

_____

Any balance or coordination problems? _____

_____

Medical History:
Family history of speech/hearing problems? _____

_____

Unusual prenatal conditions: _____

Unusual postnatal conditions: _____

Serious childhood diseases/conditions: _____

Ear infections: _____

Developmental History (age when milestones accomplished):

Sat alone: _____

Crawled: _____

Walked alone: _____

Toilet trained: _____

Speech-Language Development:

Age at first words: _____

Current speech status: _____

_____

Current language status: _____

_____

Social Development:

Is the child easily managed at home? _____

Does s/he like to play with other children? _____

What does s/he like to do most and how does s/he entertain him/herself? _____

_____

_____

Previous Treatment:

Please list the names and addresses of any physician or agency that has provided services for your child in the past:

Name	Address
_____	_____
_____	_____
_____	_____
_____	_____

Audiometer

An audiometer is the primary instrument used by the audiologist to measure hearing threshold and by the speech-language pathologist to screen for hearing loss. Audiometers vary from the simple, inexpensive screening devices used in schools and public health programs to the more elaborate and expensive diagnostic audiometers found in hospitals and clinics. Certain basic components, however, are common to all audiometers. Figure 5.1 shows an example of one of these basic units. A frequency selector dial permits selection of different pure-tone frequencies. Ordinarily, these frequencies are available at octave intervals ranging from 125 to 8,000 Hz. An interrupter switch or presentation button allows presentation of the tone to the listener. A hearing level dial controls the intensity of the signal. Most audiometers can deliver signals spanning a 100-dB range in 5-dB steps. An output selector determines whether the pure tone will be presented to the earphones for air conduction testing (for either the right or the left ear) or whether the tone is to be sent to a bone vibrator for bone conduction testing. Many audiometers also have a masking level dial, which controls the intensity of the masking noise presented to the nontest ear when masking is necessary. The more elaborate diagnostic audiometers not only can generate masking noise and pure-tone signals but also provide a means for measuring the understanding of speech signals.

Audiogram

The audiogram is a chart used to graphically record the hearing thresholds and other test results. Figure 5.2 shows an example of an audiogram and the associated symbol system recommended by the American Speech-Language-Hearing Association. The audiogram is shown in graphic form, with the signal frequencies (in hertz) displayed on the x axis and the hearing level (in decibels) represented on the y axis. The graph is designed in such a manner that the length representing 1 octave in frequency on the horizontal scale is equal in size to the length representing 20-dB hearing level on the vertical scale.

The horizontal line at the 0-dB hearing level (HL) represents normal hearing sensitivity for the average young adult. However, as described in Chapter 4, the human ear does not perceive sound equally well at all frequencies. Recall that the ear is most sensitive to sound in the intermediate-frequency region from 1,000 to 4,000 Hz and is less sensitive at both the higher and lower frequencies. Greater sound pressure is needed to elicit a threshold response at 250 Hz than at 2,000 Hz in normal ears. The audiometer is calibrated to correct for these differences in threshold sensitivity at various frequencies. Consequently, when the hearing level dial is set at zero for a given frequency,

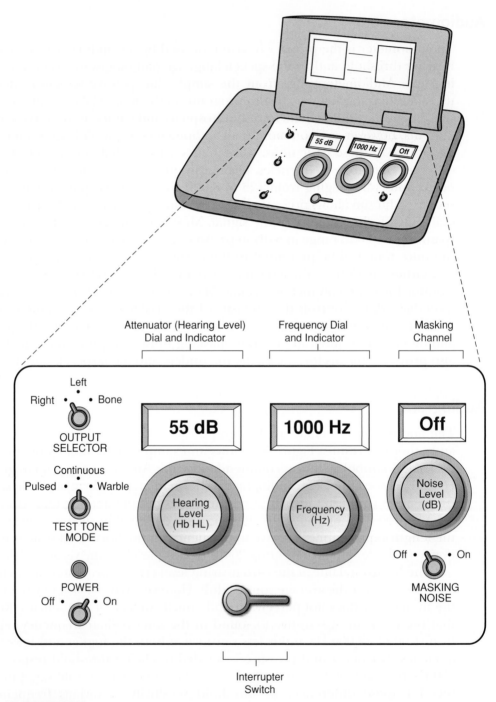

FIGURE 5.1 The basic components seen on the control panel of a pure-tone audiometer.

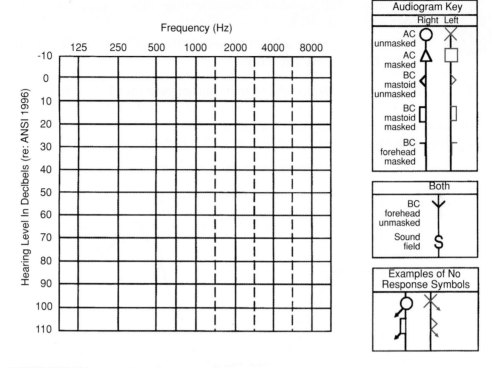

FIGURE 5.2   *Left,* Audiogram used for plotting pure-tone air and bone conduction thresholds. *Right,* The Audiogram Key displays the symbols commonly used in audiograms. *AC,* air conduction; *BC,* bone conduction.

the signal is automatically presented at the normal threshold sound pressure level required for the average young adult to hear that particular frequency (Vignette 5.2).

Results plotted on the audiogram can be used to classify the extent of a hearing impairment. This information plays a valuable role in determining the habilitative or rehabilitative needs of an individual with impaired hearing. Classification schemes using the pure-tone audiogram are based on the fact that there is a strong relationship between the threshold for those frequencies known to be important for hearing speech (500, 1,000, and 2,000 Hz) and the lowest level at which speech can be recognized accurately 50% of the time. The latter measure is generally referred to as the speech recognition threshold (SRT). Given the pure-tone thresholds at 500, 1,000, and 2,000 Hz, one can estimate the hearing loss for speech and the potential handicapping effects of the impairment. This is done by simply calculating the average (mean) loss of

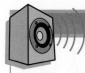

VIGNETTE 5.2 CONCEPTUAL DEMO

ILLUSTRATION OF THE RELATIONSHIP BETWEEN DECIBELS SPL (dB SPL) AND DECIBELS HL (dB HL)

The accompanying figure depicts the relationship between the dB HL scale and the dB SPL scale of sound intensity. The circles in the upper panel are the data for hearing thresholds of normal-hearing young adults. The triangles in the upper panel are hearing thresholds obtained from an individual with a high-frequency hearing loss. Note

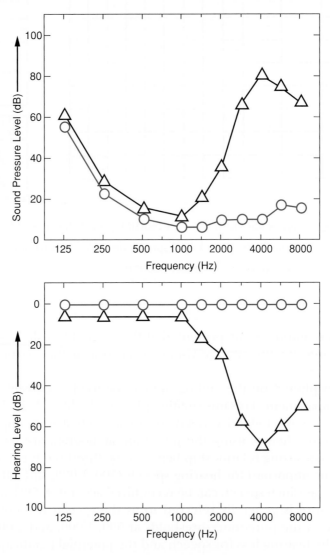

that increasing hearing loss is indicated by higher sound pressure levels at threshold. At 4000 Hz, for example, the average threshold for normal-hearing young adults is 10 dB SPL; the patient's threshold is 80 dB SPL, indicating a hearing loss of 70 dB. These same data have been replotted on the dB HL scale in the lower panel. Note now that the normal hearing threshold has been set to 0 dB HL on this scale at all frequencies. Increasing intensity is shown in a downward direction on the audiogram. Note also that the threshold for the hearing-impaired subject at 4,000 Hz is 70 dB HL. This threshold value itself then directly indicates the magnitude of hearing loss relative to normal hearing. There is no need to subtract the normal-hearing threshold value from the value observed in the impaired ear, as was the case for the dB SPL scale.

hearing for these three frequencies. This average is referred to as the three-frequency pure-tone average. Figure 5.3 shows an example of a typical classification system based on the pure-tone average. This scheme, adapted from several other systems, reflects the different classifications of hearing loss as well as the likely effects of the hearing loss on an individual's ability to hear speech. The hearing loss classes, ranging from mild to profound, are based on the pure-tone average at 500, 1,000, and 2,000 Hz. The classification of normal limits extends to 25 dB HL, and hearing levels within this range have typically been thought to produce essentially no problems with even faint speech. Some evidence indicates, however, that losses from 15 to 25 dB HL can have negative effects educationally on children. Children with hearing loss in this range should be considered for relatively unobtrusive ways to amplify the teacher's speech in the classroom that will also provide benefit to children with normal hearing in the same classroom (Chapter 6).

Measurement of Hearing

In pure-tone audiometry, thresholds are obtained by both air conduction and bone conduction. In air conduction measurement, the different pure-tone
stimuli are transmitted through earphones. The signal travels through the ear #7
canal, across the middle ear cavity via the three ossicles to the cochlea, and to the auditory central nervous system, as reviewed in Chapter 4. Air conduction thresholds reflect the integrity of the total auditory mechanism. When a person exhibits a hearing loss by air conduction, it is not possible to determine the
location of the pathology along the auditory pathway. The hearing loss could #8
be the result of (a) a problem in the outer or middle ear, (b) a difficulty at the level of the cochlea, (c) damage along the neural pathways to the brain, or (d)

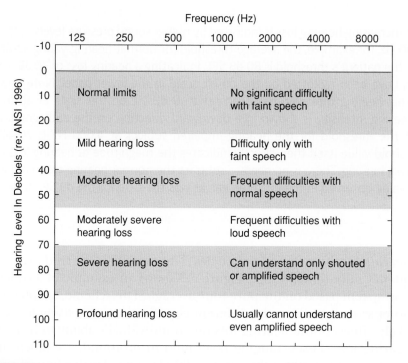

FIGURE 5.3   Classification of hearing impairment in relation to disability for speech recognition.

some combination of these. When air conduction measurements are combined with bone conduction measurements, however, it is possible to differentiate outer and middle ear problems (conductive hearing loss) from inner ear problems (sensorineural hearing loss).

In bone conduction measurement, signals are transmitted via a bone vibrator that is usually placed on the mastoid prominence of the skull (a bony prominence located behind the pinna, slightly above the level of the concha). The forehead is another position for placement of the bone vibrator. A signal transduced through the vibrator causes the skull to vibrate. The pure tone directly stimulates the cochlea, which is embedded in the skull, effectively bypassing the outer ear and middle ear systems. If an individual exhibits a reduction in hearing sensitivity when tested by air conduction yet shows normal sensitivity by bone conduction, the impairment is probably a result of an obstruction or blockage of the outer or middle ear. This condition is referred to as a conductive hearing loss. Figure 5.4 gives an audiometric example of a young child with a conductive hearing loss caused by middle ear disease. The

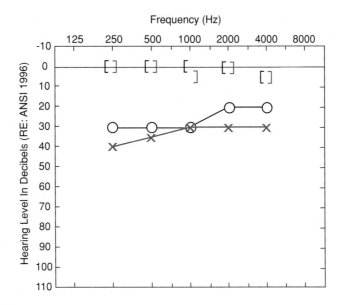

FIGURE 5.4 Pure-tone audiogram demonstrating the relation between air and bone conduction thresholds typifying mild conductive hearing impairment. Bone conduction thresholds: [, right ear;], left ear. Air conduction thresholds: O-O, right ear; X-X, left ear.

bone conduction thresholds appear close to 0 dB HL for all test frequencies. Such a finding implies that the inner ear responds to sound at normal threshold levels. The air conduction thresholds, on the other hand, are much greater than 0 dB HL. Greater sound intensity is needed for this child to hear the air-conducted pure-tone signals than is required by the average normal hearer. Because the bone conduction thresholds suggest that the inner ear is normal, the loss displayed by air conduction must result from a conductive lesion affecting the outer or middle ear.

The difference between the air conduction threshold and the bone conduction threshold at a given frequency is generally referred to as the *air-bone gap*. In Figure 5.4, for example, at 250 Hz there is a 30-dB air-bone gap in the right ear and a 40-dB gap in the left ear. Conductive hearing loss is especially prevalent among preschool and young school-aged children who experience repeated episodes of otitis media (middle-ear infection). Other examples of pathologic conditions, known to produce conductive hearing loss, include congenital atresia (absence of ear canals), blockage or occlusion of the ear canal (possibly by cerumen or earwax), perforation or scarring of the tympanic membrane, ossicular chain disruption, and otosclerosis (bony growth fixing the stapes to the oval window).

As we noted, hearing thresholds better than a hearing level of 25 dB HL are considered normal. Air-bone gaps of 10 dB or more, however, represent a significant conductive hearing loss and may require medical referral, even if the air conduction thresholds are less than 25 dB at all frequencies. That is, such small air-bone gaps, although likely to have only a marginal impact on communication, may reflect an underlying medical condition that requires follow-up examination.

A sensorineural hearing loss is suggested when the air conduction thresholds *and* bone conduction thresholds are approximately the same (within 5 dB) at all test frequencies and outside the normal limits. Sensorineural hearing impairment may be either congenital or acquired. Some of the congenital causes include heredity, complications of maternal viral and bacterial infections, and birth trauma. Factors producing acquired sensorineural hearing loss include noise, aging, inflammatory diseases (e.g., measles or mumps), and ototoxic drugs (e.g., aminoglycoside antibiotics). Figure 5.5 gives three different examples of sensorineural hearing impairment. Figure 5.5A shows the audiogram of an adult with hearing loss resulting from the use of ototoxic antibiotics. This audiogram displays a moderate bilateral sensorineural impairment with greater hearing loss in the high-frequency region. Figure 5.5B shows the audiogram of a child whose hearing impairment resulted from maternal rubella (measles). It can be seen that the magnitude of this hearing loss falls in the profound category in the region of the most critical frequencies for hearing speech (500 to 2,000 Hz). In fact, the loss is so severe that bone conduction responses could not be obtained at the maximum output of the audiometer at all test frequencies. This is indicated by the downward-pointing arrows attached to the audiometric symbols and should not be mistaken for an air-bone gap. Air conduction thresholds also could not be obtained at frequencies above 1,000 Hz because the hearing loss was so great.

The majority of sensorineural hearing losses are characterized by audiometric configurations that are flat, trough-shaped, or slightly to steeply sloping in the high frequencies. The latter is probably the most common configuration associated with acquired sensorineural hearing loss. Occasionally, however, patients display a sensorineural hearing loss in which the greatest hearing loss occurs at low and intermediate frequencies, with normal or near-normal hearing sensitivity at the high frequencies. Figure 5.5C shows an example of a typical low-frequency hearing loss. Low-tone hearing loss most commonly results from either some types of hereditary deafness or Ménière's disease. Young children whose audiograms display low-frequency hearing impairment are difficult to identify and are sometimes the unfortunate victims of misdiagnosis.

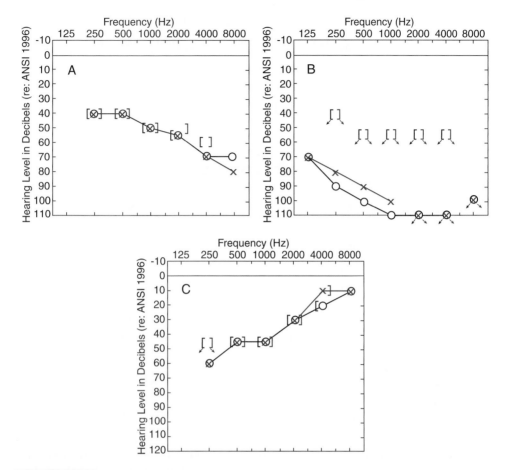

FIGURE 5.5 Three pure-tone air and bone conduction audiograms. *A,* Moderate bilateral sensorineural hearing loss. *B,* Profound bilateral sensorineural hearing loss. *C,* Low-frequency bilateral sensorineural hearing loss.

Because of their near-normal hearing sensitivity in the high frequencies, these children may respond to whispered speech and broadband stimuli at low intensity levels. In addition, unlike children with a high-frequency hearing loss, their articulation of speech is usually good. These manifestations are not typical of sensorineural hearing loss in children, which makes them more prone to misdiagnosis.

When both air conduction thresholds and bone conduction thresholds are reduced in sensitivity, but bone conduction yields better results than air conduction, the term "mixed hearing loss" is used, meaning the patient's hearing

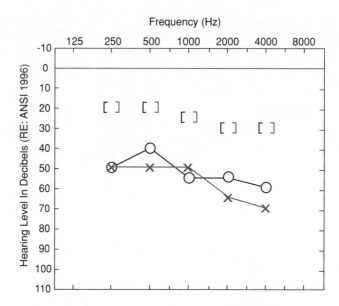

FIGURE 5.6 Pure-tone audiogram demonstrating the relation between air and bone conduction thresholds indicating a mixed (conductive and sensorineural) type of hearing loss.

loss is partially conductive and partially sensorineural. Figure 5.6 shows an audiogram depicting mixed hearing loss. Even though hearing loss is evident both for bone and air conduction thresholds, bone conduction sensitivity is consistently better across all test frequencies. This suggests that there has been some damage to the hair cells or nerve endings in the inner ear, causing a reduction in bone conduction thresholds, which is added to the reduction in air conduction thresholds resulting from malfunction of the outer ear or middle ear.

Vignette 5.3 provides a little more detail about the mechanisms underlying air conduction and bone conduction hearing tests. Additional explanation of the interpretation of thresholds from air conduction and bone conduction testing for the purpose of pinpointing the location of the pathology in the auditory periphery is also provided.

In summary, the pure-tone audiogram provides a lot of information to the audiologist regarding the location of the impairment in the periphery (conductive: outer or middle ear; sensorineural: inner ear; mixed: both), the severity of the resulting hearing loss (mild to profound), the configuration of the hearing loss (rising, flat, or sloping), and whether one or both ears are

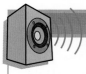

MECHANISMS UNDERLYING AIR-CONDUCTION AND BONE-CONDUCTION THRESHOLDS

This series of panels is designed to better explain the nature of hearing thresholds obtained by air conduction and by bone conduction. Panel A, for example, schematically shows the sound wave and resulting mechanical energy traveling from the outer

A. Air-conduction pathway

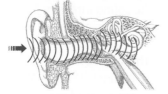

B. Bone-conduction pathway

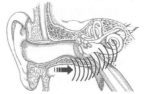

C. Outer ear damage- Higher Air-conduction threshold

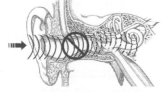

D. Outer ear damage - Normal Bone-conduction threshold

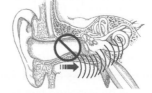

E. Middle ear damage- Higher Air-conduction threshold

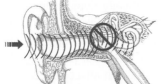

F. Middle ear damage - Normal Bone-conduction threshold

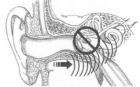

G.Inner ear damage- Higher Air-conduction threshold

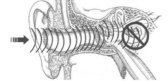

H. Inner ear damage - Higher Bone-conduction threshold

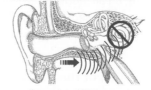

I. ME & IE damage

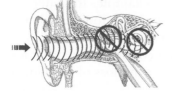

J. ME & IE damage

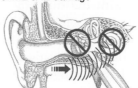

ear, through the middle ear, and mechanically stimulating the cochlea in the inner ear. Likewise, Panel B illustrates the mechanical vibration of the bony skull with a bone oscillator and a mechanical pathway directly stimulating the cochlea. The bone-conduction pathway, for the most part, can be viewed as bypassing the outer and middle ears to directly stimulate the inner ears. (B*oth* cochleas are stimulated through skull vibration.) The symbol in the next panels C and D, E and F, represents the location of pathology in the outer ear (C & D) and middle ear (E & F). Clearly, the pathology in these two areas would have a negative impact on the transmission of mechanical energy through the normal air-conduction pathway. To get through the blockage posed by the pathology in the outer or middle ear, the sound intensity for air conduction stimulation would have to be increased. In other words, a hearing loss would be measured for air conduction stimuli.

What about bone-conduction stimulation in the case of outer or middle ear pathology? This situation is illustrated schematically in Panels D and F. The mechanical bone-conduction pathway is not impacted by the presence of outer ear or middle ear pathologies and bone-conduction hearing is essentially normal. Consequently, air-conduction thresholds reveal elevated hearing thresholds and bone-conduction thresholds do not, which results in an air-bone gap.

Now, consider the case of inner ear pathology as shown in Panels G and H. Notice that the inner ear pathology occurs at the end of both the air conduction and bone conduction pathways. As a result, hearing threshold for both air and bone conduction stimulation will be impaired by the same amount. In other words, both thresholds will show the same amount of hearing loss and, as a result, there will be no air-bone gap.

Finally, the bottom two panels (I and J) schematically depict the situation for a mixed hearing loss with pathology present in both the middle ear and inner ear. The air-conduction pathway (I) is negatively impacted by both pathologies, whereas the bone-conduction pathway (J) is only affected by the inner ear pathology. As a result, bone-conduction thresholds will be higher than normal, but air-conduction thresholds, having to surmount both the middle ear and inner ear pathology will be even higher. In other words, an air-bone gap will exist and the bone conduction thresholds will indicate the presence of sensorineural (inner ear) hearing loss.

affected. Each of these factors can contribute to a breakdown in the communication chain. The implications of the findings from pure-tone audiometry also vary with the outcome obtained. For example, in general, conductive hearing loss poses a lesser threat to the communication chain because it is typically milder in degree and is often medically treatable and, as a result, will often be of short duration. An unresolved conductive hearing loss, one that becomes long lasting, or a sensorineural hearing loss of the same degree can have much greater impact on the communication chain and its development. Thus, clearly establishing the location of a peripheral problem in the outer, middle, or inner ear is crucial. The audiologist, however, routinely relies on more than just pure-tone audiometry to make this determination.

SPEECH AUDIOMETRY

The acoustic signals critical to communication are speech sounds, not the pure tones used in pure-tone audiometry. Therefore, the audiologist also assesses the impact of the hearing loss on speech communication as well. This is referred to as **speech audiometry** and additional equipment (a speech audiometer) is needed for such measurements. Typically, the audiologist makes use of a diagnostic audiometer, which includes capability for both pure-tone and speech audiometry in the same device. The speech audiometer is used to obtain two types of measurements: (a) speech recognition threshold, which corresponds to the softest level at which speech can be recognized with 50% accuracy; and (b) speech recognition score, which corresponds to the percentage of speech that can be understood when presented at sound levels well above the softest that can be heard (sound levels close to the optimal level for a given hearing impairment).

Assessment of Speech Recognition Threshold

Speech recognition threshold is the intensity at which an individual can identify simple speech materials approximately 50% of the time. It is included in the basic hearing evaluation for two specific reasons. First, it serves as an excellent check on the validity of pure-tone thresholds. There is a strong correlation between the average of the pure-tone thresholds obtained at the frequencies known to be important for speech (i.e., 500, 1,000, and 2,000 Hz) and the SRT. Large discrepancies between the SRT and this pure-tone average (PTA) may suggest functional, or nonorganic, hearing loss. A second important reason for including the SRT in the hearing evaluation is that it provides a basis for selecting the sound level at which a patient's speech recognition abilities should be tested. Finally, besides its use in the basic hearing evaluation, the SRT is also useful in the determination of functional gain in the hearing aid evaluation process.

#11

The most popular test materials used by audiologists to measure SRT are spondaic words. Spondaic words are two-syllable words spoken with equal stress on each syllable (e.g., baseball, hotdog, cowboy). A carrier phrase, such as "say the word," may precede each stimulus item.

Assessment of Suprathreshold Speech Recognition

Although the speech threshold provides the clinician with an index of the degree of hearing loss for speech, it does not offer any information regarding a person's ability to make distinctions among the various acoustic cues in our spoken language at conversational intensity levels. Unlike the situation with the SRT, attempts to calculate a person's ability to understand speech presented at comfortably loud levels based on data from the pure-tone audiogram have not been successful. Consequently, various suprathreshold speech recognition tests have been developed for the purpose of estimating a person's ability to understand speech. Three of the more common types of speech recognition tests are phonetically balanced lists of single-syllable words (e.g., dog, ball), multiple-choice tests comprised of rhyming single-syllable words (e.g., ball, tall, fall, and mall), and sentence tests.

The most popular stimuli used to assess speech understanding are phonetically balanced (PB) lists of single-syllable words, which is the only type we will review here. These word lists are referred to as "phonetically balanced" because the phonetic composition of all word lists in the test is equivalent and representative of everyday English speech. All of the PB word lists use an open-set response format. This is akin to a fill-in-the-blank test item, in which the set of possible responses is potentially unlimited and is restricted only by the listener's vocabulary. In contrast, a closed-response format is akin to a multiple-choice test item, in which the listener is presented with a set of several alternative responses for each test item, one of which is the monosyllabic word spoken by the examiner. A typical presentation includes the use of a carrier phrase, such as "Say the word. . . ." For example, a typical sequence might be "Say the word *dog*" (the patient responds), "Say the word *ball*" (the patient responds), and so on. Typically, the instruction to the patient is simply to repeat aloud the last word heard for each test item ("dog" and "ball" in the preceding two examples).

The procedures used to obtain SRT and speech recognition scores are standardized for adults so that similar results can be obtained from clinic to clinic or from time to time for the same patient in the same clinic. There are also variations of all of these procedures, as well as for pure-tone audiometry, for use with children of various ages. The details of these adaptations are not included here. In the end, the audiologist uses a variety of age-appropriate techniques to get the best estimate of hearing for pure tones and hearing for speech from the patient and records these on the audiogram.

Pure-tone and speech-audiometry, however, involve voluntary behavioral responses from the patient. As with any such measurements, there can be variability or error in the measurements and this, in turn, can impact the certainty of the diagnosis. As a result, audiologists have developed other complementary measurements that assess the auditory system, but do not require behavioral responses from the patient. These can be especially valuable in the assessment of young children who may be more variable in their behavioral responses. One set of complementary measurements has become a standard part of the basic audiologic test battery and is known as "acoustic immittance measurement."

ACOUSTIC IMMITTANCE MEASUREMENT

When an acoustic wave strikes the eardrum of the normal ear, a portion of the signal is transmitted through the middle ear to the cochlea, while the remaining part of the wave is reflected back out the external canal. The reflected energy forms a sound wave traveling in an outward direction with an amplitude and phase that depend on the opposition encountered at the tympanic membrane. The energy of the reflected wave is greatest when the middle ear system is stiff or immobile, as in such pathologic conditions as otitis media with effusion and otosclerosis. On the other hand, an ear with ossicular-chain dislocation or interruption will reflect considerably less sound back into the canal because of the reduced stiffness. A greater portion of the acoustic wave will be transmitted to the middle ear under these circumstances. The reflected sound wave, therefore, carries information about the status of the middle ear system.

Impedance is the term used to describe the opposition to flow of acoustic (mechanical) energy through the middle ear. The reciprocal of impedance is admittance. An ear with high impedance has low admittance and vice versa. Admittance describes the relative ease with which energy flows through a system, such as the middle ear. Some commercially available devices used by the clinician measure quantities related to acoustic impedance of the middle ear, whereas others measure quantities related to acoustic admittance. In an effort to provide a common vocabulary for results obtained with either device, professionals have decided to use the term "immittance." Immittance itself is not a physical quantity, but simply a term that can be used to refer to either impedance data or admittance data.

The measurement of **acoustic immittance** at the tympanic membrane is an important component of the basic hearing evaluation. This sensitive and objective diagnostic tool has been used to identify the presence of fluid in the middle ear, to evaluate eustachian tube and facial nerve function, to predict audiometric findings, to determine the nature of hearing loss, and to assist in diagnosing the site of auditory lesion. This technique is considered particularly useful in the assessment of difficult-to-test persons, including very young children.

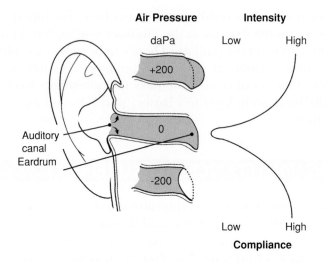

FIGURE 5.7 Concepts of immittance applied in practice. The middle column shows three different air pressures developed in the ear canal (−200, 0, and +200 daPa), and the dotted line in the drawings at the top and bottom of this column represent the resting position of the eardrum (at 0 daPa). The right column shows both the sound intensity of the probe tone recorded in the ear canal as the air pressure is changed from −200 daPa (top) to +200 daPa (bottom) and the corresponding changes in the compliance of the middle ear.

Figure 5.7 shows how this concept may be applied to actual practice. A pliable probe tip is inserted carefully into the ear canal and an airtight seal is obtained so that varying amounts of air pressure can be applied to the ear cavity by pumping air into the ear canal or suctioning it out. A positive amount of air pressure (usually +200 daPa)* is then introduced into the airtight ear canal, forcing the tympanic membrane inward. The eardrum is now stiffer than it is in its natural state because of the positive pressure created in the ear canal. A low-frequency pure tone is then introduced, and a tiny microphone measures the level of the sound reflected from the stiffened eardrum. A low-frequency tone is used because this is the frequency region most affected by changes in stiffness (Chapter 2). Keeping the intensity of the probe tone introduced into the ear

---

*A daPa is a measure of air pressure in units of decapascals. 1 daPa = 10 Pa = 1.02 mm H_2O. Millimeters (mm) H_2O refers to the amount of pressure to push a column of water in a special tube to a given height in millimeters. For measurements of immittance, air pressure is generally expressed relative to ambient air pressure. That is, ambient air pressure is represented as 0 daPa, and a pressure of 100 daPa above ambient pressure is represented as +100 daPa.

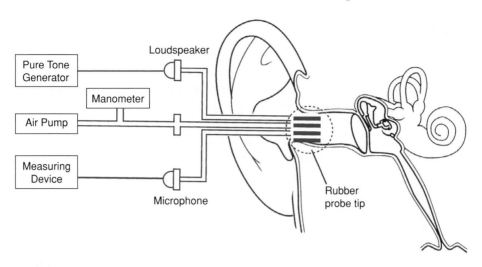

FIGURE 5.8 Components of an immittance instrument.

canal constant, the pressure is then reduced slowly, causing the tympanic membrane to become more compliant (less stiff). As the tympanic membrane becomes increasingly compliant, more of the acoustic signal will be passed through the middle ear, and the level of the reflected sound in the ear canal will decrease. When the air pressure in the ear canal equals the air pressure in the middle ear, the tympanic membrane will move with the greatest ease. As the pressure is reduced further, the tympanic membrane is pulled outward, and the eardrum again becomes less mobile. As before, when the eardrum becomes stiffer or less compliant, more low-frequency energy is reflected off the tympanic membrane, and the sound level within the ear canal increases.

Figure 5.8 illustrates the basic components of most immittance instruments. The probe tip is sealed in the ear canal, providing a closed cavity. The probe contains three small ports that are connected to: (a) a sound source that generates a low-frequency (usually 220 or 660 Hz) pure tone; (b) a microphone to measure the reflected sound wave; and (c) an air pump and manometer for varying the air pressure within the ear canal.

IMMITTANCE TEST BATTERY

Three basic measurements—tympanometry, static acoustic immittance, and threshold of the acoustic reflex—commonly make up the basic acoustic immittance test battery.

Tympanometry

Acoustic immittance at the tympanic membrane of a normal ear changes systematically as air pressure in the external canal is varied above and below ambient air pressure (Fig. 5.7). The normal relationship between air pressure changes and changes in immittance is frequently altered in the presence of middle ear disease. Tympanometry is the measurement of the mobility of the middle ear when air pressure in the external canal is varied from +200 to −400 daPa. Results from tympanometry are then plotted on a graph, with air pressure along the x axis and immittance, or *compliance*, along the y axis.[†] Figure 5.9 illustrates some of the tympanograms commonly seen in normal and pathologic ears.

Various estimates have been made of the air pressure in the ear canal that results in the least amount of reflected sound energy from normal middle ears. This air pressure is routinely referred to as the *peak pressure point*. A normal tympanogram for an adult (Fig. 5.9A) has a peak pressure point between −100 and +40 daPa, which suggests that the middle ear functions optimally at or near ambient pressure (0 daPa). Tympanograms that peak at a point ≤−150 daPa (Fig. 5.9B) suggest malfunction of the middle ear pressure-equalizing system. This malfunction might be a result of eustachian tube malfunction, early or resolving serous otitis media, or acute otitis media. (These and other disorders were described in Chapter 4.) Ears that contain fluid behind the eardrum are characterized by a flat tympanogram at a high impedance or low admittance value without a peak pressure point (Fig. 5.9C). This implies an excessively stiff system that does not allow for an increase in sound transmission through the middle ear under any pressure state. The amplitude (height) of the tympanogram also provides information about the compliance or elasticity of the system. A stiff middle ear (as in, for example, ossicular-chain fixation) is represented by a shallow amplitude, suggesting high acoustic impedance or low admittance (Fig. 5.9D). Conversely, an ear with abnormally low acoustic impedance or high admittance (as in an interrupted ossicular chain or a hypermobile tympanic membrane) is revealed by a tympanogram with a very high amplitude (Fig. 5.9E).

Flat tympanograms can also be observed when the probe tip of the immittance device is blocked (for example, with earwax) or when there is a perforation of the eardrum. In these cases, when the shape of the tympanogram is the same

---

[†]Throughout this text, we have assumed that immittance measurements are made with an impedance meter. With such a device, immittance values are described in arbitrary units, frequently labeled "compliance." These devices do not actually measure compliance.

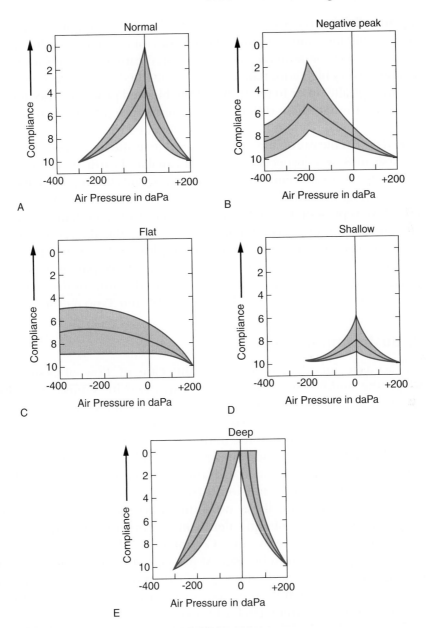

FIGURE 5.9 Tympanometric configurations for normal and pathologic ears are shown. Measured tympmanograms falling in the *blue shaded regions* would be classified using the label at the top of each tympanogram (normal, negative peak, flat, etc.).

(flat), the clinician relies on differences in the overall amplitude of the impedance or admittance value. A blocked probe tip, for example, will show a very high impedance (very low admittance), a perforated eardrum often shows a very low impedance (very high admittance), and a fluid-filled middle ear is somewhere in between, typically closer to the values of the blocked probe tip. Because the tympanograms are flat, these differences in immittance amplitude manifest themselves at the initial reading of immittance obtained with a high positive pressure (+200 daPa); a measurement often referred to as the *equivalent ear canal volume.* Of course, otoscopic inspection of the ear canal and eardrum can help differentiate among these different causes for tympanograms having flat shape too.

#13

Tympanograms are frequently labeled as types. Type A tympanograms (Fig. 5.9A) represent normal tympanograms (normal shape, peak-pressure point, and amplitude), Type B tympanograms are flat (Fig. 5.9C), and Type C tympanograms have normal shape and amplitude, but a negative peak-pressure point (Fig. 5.9B). Two subtypes of Type A tympanograms, which are abnormal only with regard to the peak amplitude and not the shape or peak-pressure point, are Type A_s (shallow; Fig. 5.9D) and Type A_d (deep; Fig. 5.9E).

Static Acoustic Immittance

Static acoustic immittance measures the ease of flow of acoustic energy through the middle ear and is usually expressed in "equivalent volume" in cubic centimeters. To obtain this measurement, immittance is first determined under a positive pressure (+200 daPa) artificially induced in the canal. Very little sound is admitted through the middle ear under this extreme positive pressure, with much of the acoustic energy reflected back into the ear canal. Next, a similar determination is made with the eardrum in its most compliant position, thus maximizing transmission through the middle ear cavity. The arithmetic difference between these two immittance values, usually recorded in cubic centimeters (cm^3) of equivalent volume, provides an estimate of immittance at the tympanic membrane. Compliance values less than or equal to 0.25 cm^3 of equivalent volume suggest low acoustic immittance (indicative of stiffening pathologies), and values greater than or equal to 2.0 cm^3 generally indicate abnormally high immittance (suggestive of ossicular discontinuity or healed tympanic membrane perforations).

Acoustic Reflex Threshold

The acoustic reflex threshold is defined as the lowest possible intensity needed to elicit a contraction of the muscles in the middle ear. Contraction of the middle ear muscles, evoked by intense sound, results in a temporary increase in

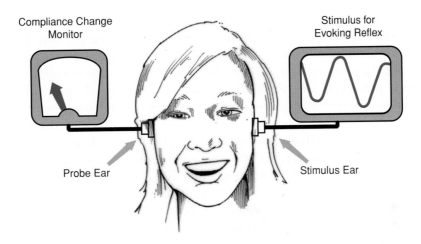

Compliance Change Monitor

Stimulus for Evoking Reflex

Probe Ear

Stimulus Ear

FIGURE 5.10 Example of how an acoustic reflex is obtained for contralateral stimulus presentation. Essentially, for ipsilateral measurements, the functions of the probe tip and the earphone are combined so that the reflex-eliciting stimulus and the immittance change that results from the muscle contraction can be measured in the same ear.

the middle ear impedance. The acoustic reflex is a consensual phenomenon; acoustic stimulation to one ear will elicit a muscle contraction and subsequent impedance change in both ears. Often, the acoustic reflex is monitored in the ear canal contralateral to the ear receiving the sound stimulus. Figure 5.10 shows how it is measured. A headphone is placed on one ear, and the probe assembly is inserted into the contralateral (opposite) ear. When the signal transduced from the earphone reaches an intensity sufficient to evoke an acoustic reflex, the stiffness of the middle ear is increased in both ears. This results in more sound being reflected from the eardrum, and a subsequent increase in sound pressure is observed on the immittance instrument. In recording the data, it is standard procedure to consider the ear stimulated with the intense sound as the ear under test. Because the ear stimulated is contralateral to the ear in which the reflex is measured, these reflex thresholds are referred to as *contralateral reflex thresholds*. It is also frequently possible to present the loud reflex-activating stimulus through the probe assembly itself. In this case, the reflex is both activated and measured in the same ear. This is referred to as an *ipsilateral acoustic reflex*.

#14

In the normal ear, contraction of middle ear muscles occurs with pure tones ranging from 65 to 95 dB HL. A conductive hearing loss, however, tends to either elevate or eliminate the reflex response. When acoustic reflex information is used in conjunction with tympanometry and static acoustic immittance measurements, it serves to further substantiate the existence of a middle ear disorder. With unilateral conductive hearing loss, failure to elicit the reflex depends on the size of the air-bone gap and on the ear in which the probe tip is inserted. If the stimulus is presented to the good ear and the probe tip is placed on the affected side, an air-bone gap of only 10 dB will usually abolish the reflex response. In this case, the pathology present in the "probe ear" has increased the stiffness of the middle ear so much that small increases in stiffness associated with the acoustic reflex either do not occur or cannot be measured. If, however, the stimulus is presented to the pathologic ear and the probe is in the normal ear, a gap of 25 dB is needed to abolish or significantly elevate the reflex threshold. In this case, the contralateral acoustic reflex is absent because the middle-ear pathology decreases the amplitude of the reflex-activating sound reaching the cochlea to levels that are too soft to elicit the reflex.

Acoustic reflex thresholds can also be useful in differentiating whether a sensorineural hearing loss is caused by a lesion in the inner ear or to one in the auditory nerve. For hearing losses ranging from mild to severe, the acoustic reflex threshold is more likely to be elevated or absent in ears with neural pathology than in those with cochlear damage. The pattern of acoustic reflex thresholds for ipsilateral and contralateral stimulation across both ears, moreover, can aid in diagnosing brainstem lesions affecting the reflex pathways in the auditory brainstem.

Immittance can be most valuable in the assessment of young children, although it does have some diagnostic limitations. Further, although electro-acoustic immittance measures are ordinarily simple and quick to obtain, special considerations and skills are required to obtain these measures successfully from infants. Variation in test stimuli, such as the use of higher frequency, might also be needed to ensure valid results. Immittance measures in young children might be confined to handheld immittance screeners that enable quick measurement of tympanograms and ipsilateral acoustic reflexes at a single high intensity (often at a single frequency too, such as 1000 Hz).

Although immittance tests may be administered to neonates and young infants with a reasonable amount of success, tympanometry may have limited value with children younger than 7 months of age. Below this age, there is a poor correlation between tympanometry and the actual condition of the middle ear. In very young infants, a normal tympanogram does not necessarily imply that there is a normal middle ear system. However, a flat tympanogram obtained in an infant strongly suggests a diseased ear. Consequently, it is still worthwhile to administer immittance tests to this population.

Another limitation of immittance measurements is the difficulty of obtaining measurements from a hyperactive child or a child who is crying, yawning, or continually talking. A young child who exhibits excessive body movement or head turning will make it almost impossible to maintain an airtight seal with the probe tip. Vocalization produces middle ear muscle activity that, in turn, causes continual alterations in the compliance of the tympanic membrane, making immittance measurements impossible. With difficult-to-test and younger children, specialized techniques are needed to keep the child relatively calm and quiet. For young children, it is always recommended that a second person be involved in the evaluation. While the child is sitting on the parent's lap, one person can place the earphone and insert the probe tip and a second person can manipulate the controls of the equipment. With infants below 2 years of age, placing the earphones and headband on the child's head is often distracting. It may be helpful to remove the earphone from the headband, rest the band over the mother's shoulder, and insert the probe tip into the child's ear. It is also helpful to use some distractive techniques that will occupy the child's attention during the test (Vignette 5.4).

Basic Audiologic Test Battery

In the measurement of auditory function, the most meaningful information can be gleaned only when the entire test battery of pure-tone and speech audiometry together with immittance measurements is used. If just one or two of these procedures are used, valuable clinical information will be lost because each of these clinical tools offers a unique and informative set of data. In particular, the reader should keep in mind the differences between pure-tone measures and electro-acoustic-immittance measurements. Pure-tone audiometry does not measure the immittance of the middle ear, just as immittance does not measure hearing sensitivity. Although an abnormal audiogram strongly suggests the presence of a hearing loss, abnormal immittance does not. Abnormal immittance findings in the absence of significant hearing loss, on the other hand, can be sufficient grounds for medical referral. A test-battery approach is essential. Vignettes 5.5, 5.6, and 5.7 show examples of applications of the test battery.

#23 & #24

ADDITIONAL SPECIAL TESTS

Administration of the basic audiologic test battery determines whether or not the patient has any hearing loss; what effect the hearing loss, if present, has on speech understanding; and whether the nature of the hearing loss is conductive, sensorineural, or a combination of the two (mixed). Administration of the immittance battery can also evaluate middle ear function regardless of

VIGNETTE 5.4   CLINICAL APPLICATIONS

DISTRACTIVE TECHNIQUES WHEN OBTAINING IMMITTANCE MEASURES FROM YOUNG CHILDREN

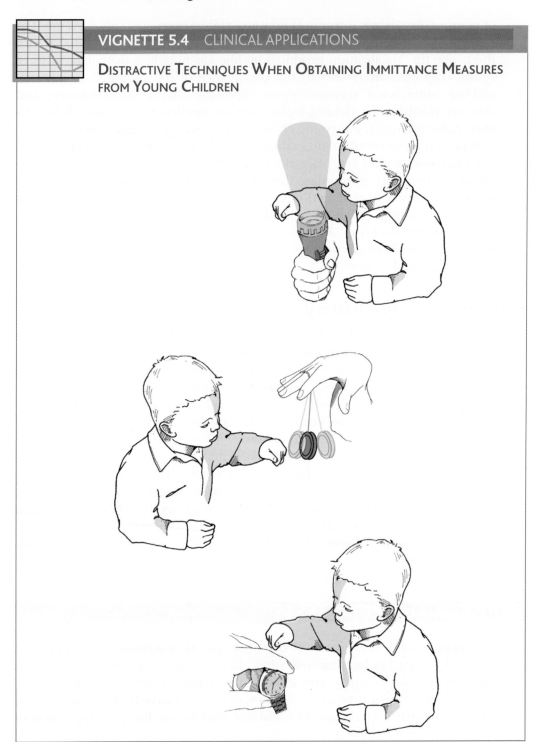

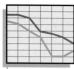

VIGNETTE 5.5 CLINICAL APPLICATIONS

A 6-Year-Old Child with Bilateral Otitis Media

The accompanying charts show a mild-to-moderate bilateral hearing loss for air conduction; bone conduction thresholds are normal in both ears. Such a discrepancy between air conduction and bone conduction thresholds suggests a conductive loss. The SRTs are compatible with the pure-tone data. Also, when the signal is made comfortably loud, suprathreshold speech recognition is excellent in both ears. Good speech recognition is consistent with a middle ear disorder. Immittance confirms the impression of a conductive loss. The light blue shaded areas on the tympanogram and static immittance forms represent normative data. The tympanograms are flat, the static immittance is well below normal, and acoustic reflexes are absent in both ears. This general pattern is consistent with a middle ear complication and strongly suggests a fluid-filled middle ear, thus requiring a medical referral. If however, there is no evidence of previous middle ear problems and the child has no complaints, a recheck should be recommended in 3 weeks. If the same results are obtained, the child should be referred to the family physician, pediatrician, or otolaryngologist.

Educationally, such a problem can be relatively serious if medical intervention does not result in a speedy return to completely normal hearing levels. Such children are likely to appear listless and inattentive in the classroom, and their performance soon begins to deteriorate. Both the teacher and the parents should receive an explanation of these probable consequences from the audiologist. In counseling the teacher, emphasis should be placed on establishing favorable classroom seating, supplementing

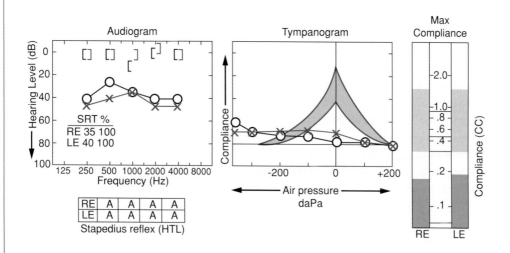

auditory input with visual cues, articulating clearly and forcefully, and frequently reiterating assignments. If the condition does not respond readily to medical treatment, amplification, along with other remedial measures such as speech reading instruction and training in listening skills, should not be ruled out. Above all, the child will need patient understanding while the hearing level is diminished and sometimes fluctuating from one day to the next.

whether a measurable hearing loss is present. Thus, through interpretation of the results from the basic audiologic test battery, the clinician can determine where in the peripheral portion of the auditory system a lesion may be located.

Additional special auditory tests are needed, however, to determine whether lesions are present in more central portions of the ascending nervous system, such as the auditory nerve, brainstem, or cortex. A patient with a life-threatening tumor affecting the auditory nerve, for example, will frequently have pure-tone test results consistent with a high-frequency sensorineural hearing loss; this is a pattern of hearing loss most frequently associated with a variety of cochlear lesions, rather than a tumor on the auditory nerve. Other components of the basic hearing test battery, however, may provide some "warning signs" suggesting that the lesion responsible for the hearing loss is affecting the auditory nerve. For example, the hearing loss in such cases usually affects the high frequencies and is different in the two ears, often leaving one ear completely unaffected. In addition, speech recognition scores in the impaired ear are often reduced much more than would be expected on the basis of the pure-tone hearing loss. Finally, acoustic reflex thresholds for the affected ear are typically elevated above the normal range (>100 dB HL). Although these features are typical for many patients with tumors affecting the auditory nerve, many cases manifest only one or two of these features. Patients with inner ear pathology, moreover, may also manifest one or more of these features.

A battery of special auditory tests has been developed to assist in the identification of lesions occurring central to the cochlea or inner ear. These lesions are referred to as *retrocochlear lesions*. Historically, this test battery was based on a variety of behavioral tests that used pure tones as stimuli. After several years of test development and refinement, most of these tests were still only 60% to 70% accurate in identifying retrocochlear impairments. Many individuals with cochlear hearing loss were falsely identified as having retrocochlear lesions, and still more retrocochlear lesions were identified as cochlear.

Today's battery of special auditory tests consists of several tests, few of which involve behavioral measurements in response to pure-tone stimulation. Detailed descriptions of these procedures are beyond the scope of this book. It is important

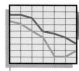

VIGNETTE 5.6   CLINICAL APPLICATIONS

AN 8-YEAR-OLD CHILD WITH BILATERAL SEVERE-TO-PROFOUND SENSORINEURAL HEARING LOSS!

The pure-tone results in the accompanying figure display a severe to profound sensorineural hearing loss. Bone conduction responses could not be obtained at the maximum output limits of the audiometer. The SRTs using selected spondees were compatible with the pure-tone data. Suprathreshold speech recognition scores could not be obtained because of the severity of the loss. Immittance results on both ears show tympanograms and static immittance values to be within the normal range. Acoustic reflexes are absent in both ears, but these usually cannot be elicited with a hearing loss in excess of 85 dB HL.

These audiologic results confirm the presence of a sensorineural hearing impairment, which is so severe that the best possible educational opportunities must be made available and, at age 8 years, will hopefully have been in place already for several years. Periodic audiologic evaluations are highly important in the optimal educational management of such children.

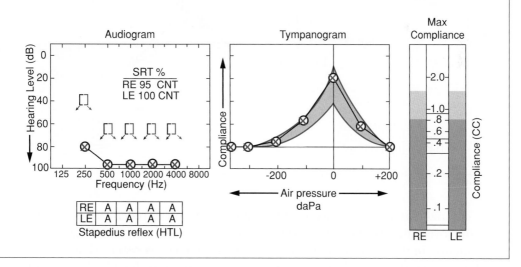

here to note only that the basic audiologic test battery is limited in its diagnostic usefulness. Additional special auditory tests can be performed in the event that any of the retrocochlear warning signs described above are found after performing the basic tests. Readers who desire to learn more about the special auditory test battery can consult the Suggested Readings at the end of this chapter.

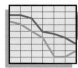

ADULT WITH A BILATERAL MILD TO MODERATE SENSORINEURAL HEARING LOSS

The pure-tone results accompanying this vignette show a bilateral sloping sensorineural hearing loss in an elderly adult. The SRTs are compatible with the pure-tone data, and suprathreshold speech recognition is only fair to good, even when the signal is made comfortably loud. Immittance results show normal tympanograms and static immittance for both ears, with acoustic reflexes present, but elevated, bilaterally.

Recommended treatment in this case would most likely be the use of two hearing aids, although there are limitations to the benefits achievable with amplification alone (Chapter 7). It may also be necessary to provide special assistance in the form of training in auditory and visual (speechreading) communication skills.

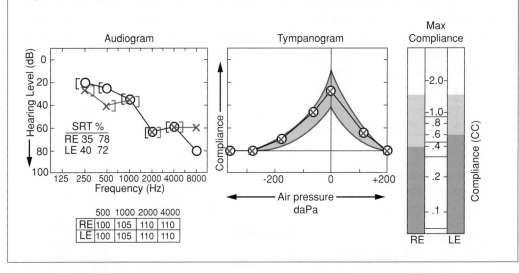

	500	1000	2000	4000
RE	100	105	110	110
LE	100	105	110	110

Finally, an area that has received much attention in recent years—much of it controversial, especially in school-age children—has been the diagnosis of dysfunction in the auditory portions of the central nervous system. These problems have generally been labeled as auditory processing disorder (APD). The reliability and validity of many of the tests developed to identify APD, in both children and adults, are still being investigated. One of the challenges has been to demonstrate that such tests are truly measuring auditory abilities and not more general cognitive function. Until such tests are developed and norms using them established, however, the diagnosis and treatment of such disorders is likely to remain controversial. (See Vignette 5.8 on the importance of test reliability and validity.)

VIGNETTE 5.8   FURTHER DISCUSSION

ILLUSTRATION OF THE IMPORTANCE OF TEST RELIABILITY AND VALIDITY

The reliability and validity of a test represents essential information that must be known before the widespread use of that test. Unfortunately, because of the pressures of solving problems for patients today, audiologists often don't feel that they have the time to wait for the needed research to be completed before the use of a newly developed test. The testing of APD in children is clearly an area that exemplifies this problem. Often, tests have been pressed into use before clearly establishing their reliability or validity as tests of APD.

In general, the reliability of the test refers to its accuracy or stability. Ideally, if the same test were administered to the same individual under identical conditions on 10 successive occasions, with no memory, learning, or fatigue involved, we would like all 10 scores to be identical. For behavioral testing of humans, especially children, however, this ideal is seldom achieved. Rather, the scores vary from test to retest because of a wide variety of factors. The greater the variation in test scores in this hypothetical scenario, the poorer the reliability of the test. Many tests of APD have been found to have unacceptable reliability. For some of the proposed APD tests, the scores can be expected to vary from test to retest such that the diagnostic disposition will likely vary from "normal" to "abnormal" (or vice versa). Clearly, such tests would be unacceptably unreliable for widespread clinical use.

Perhaps an even thornier issue, though, has to do with establishing the validity of a test. There are many kinds of test validity, but in all cases, evaluation of a test's validity attempts to determine how well the proposed test measures what it was designed to measure. In the case of APD, is the proposed test measuring "central auditory processing"? First, it must be demonstrated that poor performance on the test cannot be attributed to peripheral auditory deficits. Although this has been an infrequent problem when APD has been studied in children, it has been a very common problem when APD has been studied in the elderly. Second, it must be demonstrated that the test is sensitive to an auditory deficit and not representative of a more general cognitive problem that can affect multiple sensory modalities. Often, in this regard, clinical researchers have taken the approach that a similarity in responses implies similarity in causality. Several tests of APD, for example, make use of tasks that were validated on cases of surgically or radiologically confirmed central auditory lesions (for example, stroke patients or patients with tumors in the central pathways). When audiologists observed similar (but usually not identical) trends in performance on proposed APD tests in individuals with no known central auditory lesions, they then concluded that the locus of the dysfunction had to be central because the response pattern was similar to that obtained from patients with known central lesions.

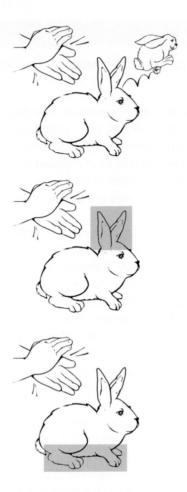

A key problem with such reasoning is shown with the fictitious "hand-clap" test of hearing illustrated here. First, the researcher establishes that normal-hearing rabbits will hop away in response to a clap of the hands (top panel). Next, a rabbit's ears are surgically destroyed. (Relax! This is just a hypothetical experiment.) The experimenter then demonstrates that the rabbit fails to hop away in response to a clap of the hands (middle panel). Thus, the test has been validated as being sensitive to the presence of a hearing impairment. Now, another rabbit's legs are surgically removed and the experimenter again claps his or her hands. The rabbit fails to hop away and the experimenter, noting the same response from those rabbits without ears, concludes that "rabbits without legs can't hear"! Clearly, the faulty reasoning in this analogy is apparent. Similarity or even equivalence of responses does not confirm similarity (or equivalence) of the underlying causal factors.

In recent years, researchers have realized the need for reliable and valid measures of APD, in both children and adults. Several tests are under development and evaluation at present and it is hoped that these tools will be available for widespread clinical use in the near future.

SUMMARY

We have reviewed the basic components of the test battery used in the measurement of auditory function. This includes the measurement of pure-tone threshold by air and bone conduction, speech audiometry, and immittance measurements. The results from these various approaches, when used as a battery, give the audiologist good insight into the nature and extent of the auditory disorder. The resulting diagnosis will also have implications for the development and use of the communication chain by the patient, as well as approaches to remedying any disruptions or breaks in the communication chain.

CHAPTER REVIEW QUESTIONS

1. Draw and label the axes of an audiogram. Shade in the region that is considered to be "normal hearing."
2. Using the audiogram you drew in Question 1, using the appropriate symbols, show a mild conductive hearing loss in the right ear. What disorder might be associated with this hearing loss?
3. Based on the audiogram you drew in Question 2 and the disorder that you associated with it, what immittance test results (tympanogram and ipsilateral acoustic reflex thresholds) would be expected for the right ear?
4. Now, draw a mild-to-severe sloping sensorineural hearing loss in the left ear, using the appropriate symbols. What disorder might be associated with the pattern of hearing loss you drew?
5. Based on the audiogram you drew in Question 4 and the hypothesized disorder associated with it, draw the tympanogram most likely to be measured and indicate the expected ipsilateral acoustic reflex thresholds.
6. Does tympanometry represent a measurement of hearing loss? That is, do individuals with abnormal tympanograms have hearing loss? Do individuals with hearing loss have abnormal tympanograms?

SUGGESTED READINGS

American Speech-Language-Hearing Association. Guidelines for audiometric symbols. *ASHA*. 1990;32(Suppl 2):25–30.

American Speech-Language-Hearing Association. Guidelines for determining threshold level for speech. *ASHA*. 1988;30(3):85–90.

Bench J, Koval A, Bamford J. The BKB (Bamford-Koval-Bench) sentence lists for partially-hearing children. *Br J Audiol*. 1979;13:108–112.

Bess FH. Clinical assessment of speech recognition. In: Konkle DF, Rintelmann WF, eds. *Principles of Speech Audiometry*. Baltimore: University Park Press; 1982.

Bess FH. The minimally hearing impaired child. *Ear Hearing*. 1985;6:43–47.

Bess FH, Chase PA, Gravel JS, et al. Amplification for infants and children with hearing loss—1995 position statement. *Am J Audiol*. 1996;5:53–68.

Bluestone CD, Beery QC, Paradise JL. Audiometry and tympanometry in relation to middle ear effusions in children. *Laryngoscope*. 1963;83:594–604.

Carhart R. Future horizons in audiological diagnosis. *Ann Otol Rhinol Laryngol*. 1968;77:706–716.

Carhart R, Jerger JF. Preferred method for clinical determination of pure-tone thresholds. *J Speech Hear Disord*. 1959;24:330–345.

Clifton RA. Development of spatial hearing. In: Werner LA, Rubel EW, eds. *Developmental Psychoacoustics.* Washington, DC: American Psychological Association; 1992.

Cox R, Alexander G, Gilmore C, Puskalich KM. Use of the Connected Speech Test (CST) with hearing-impaired listeners. *Ear Hear.* 1988;9:198–207.

Diefendorf AO. Pediatric audiology. In: Lass NJ, McReynolds LV, Northern JL, Yoder DE, eds. *Handbook of Speech-Language Pathology and Audiology.* Philadelphia: BC Decker; 1988.

Egan J. Articulation testing methods. *Laryngoscope.* 1948;58:955–991.

Haskins HA. A phonetically balanced test of speech discrimination for children. Master's thesis. Evanston, IL: Northwestern University; 1949.

Hirsh IJ, Davis H, Silverman SR, et al. Development of materials for speech audiometry. *J Speech Hear Disord.* 1952;17:321–337.

Hood JD. The principles and practice of bone-conduction audiometry: A review of the present position. *Laryngoscope.* 1960;70:1211–1228.

House AS, Williams CE, Hecker MHL, Kryter KD. Articulation testing methods: Consonantal differentiation in a closed-response set. *J Acoust Soc Am.* 1965;20:463–474.

Jerger S. Speech audiometry. In Jerger J, ed. *Pediatric Audiology.* San Diego: College Hill Press; 1984.

Jerger S, Lewis S, Hawkins J, Jerger J. Pediatric speech intelligibility test I. Generation of test materials. *Int J Pediatr Otorhinolaryngol.* 1980;2:217–230.

Kalikow DN, Stevens KN, Elliott LL. Development of a test of speech intelligibility in noise using sentence materials with controlled word predictability. *J Acoust Soc Am.* 1977;61:1337–1351.

Katz J. *Handbook of Clinical Audiology.* 6th Ed. Baltimore: Lippincott Williams & Wilkins; in press.

Katz DR, Elliott LL. Development of a new children's speech discrimination test. Paper presented at the convention of the American Speech-Language-Hearing Association. Chicago: November 18–21, 1978.

Levitt H, Resnick SB. Speech reception by the hearing impaired: Methods of testing and the development of new tests. In: Ludvigsen C, Barfod J, eds. Sensorineural Hearing Impaired and Hearing Aids. *Scand Audiol Suppl.* 1978;6:107–130.

Martin FN. Minimum effective masking levels in threshold audiometry. *J Speech Hear Disord.* 1974;39:280–285.

Northern JL. Acoustic impedance in the pediatric population. In Bess FH, ed. *Childhood Deafness: Causation, Assessment and Management.* New York: Grune & Stratton; 1977.

Northern JL, Downs MP. *Hearing in Children.* 5th Ed. Philadelphia: Lippincott Williams & Wilkins; 2001.

Olsen WO, Matkin ND. Speech audiometry. In Rintelmann WF, ed: *Hearing Assessment*. Baltimore: University Park Press; 1979.

Owens E, Schubert ED. Development of the California consonant test. *J Speech Hear Res*. 1977;20:463–474.

Ross M, Lerman J. A picture identification test for hearing impaired children. *J Speech Hear Res*. 1970;13:44–53.

Sanders JW. Masking. In Katz J, ed. *Handbook of Clinical Audiology*. 2nd Ed. Baltimore: Williams & Wilkins; 1978:124.

Sanders JW. Diagnostic audiology. In Lass NJ, McReynolds NJ, Northern JL, Yoder DE, eds. *Handbook of Speech-Language Pathology and Audiology*. Philadelphia: BC Decker; 1988.

Schwartz D, Josey AF, Bess FH, eds. Proceedings of meeting in honor of Professor Jay Sanders. *Ear Hear*. 1987;8:4.

Shanks JE, Lilly DJ, Margolis RH, Wiley TL, Wilson RH. Tympanometry. *J Speech Hear Disord*. 1988;53:354–377.

Studebaker GA. Clinical masking in air- and bone-conducted stimuli. *J Speech Hear Disord*. 1964;29:23–35.

Tharpe AM, Ashmead DH. A longitudinal investigation of infant auditory sensitivity. *Am J Audiol*. 2001;10:104–112.

Tillman TW, Olsen WO. Speech audiometry. In Jerger J, ed: *Modern Developments in Audiology*. New York: Academic Press; 1973.

Tillman TW, Carhart R. *An Expanded Test for Speech Discrimination Using CNC Monosyllabic Words*. Northwestern University Auditory Test No. 6. Technical Report No. SAM-TR-66-55. Brooks Air Force Base, TX: USAF School of Aerospace Medicine; 1966.

CHAPTER 6

Screening for Hearing Loss and Middle Ear Status

CHAPTER OBJECTIVES

- To recognize the importance of screening as a tool to identify possible cases of hearing loss or middle ear pathology as the first step toward treatment;
- To understand the principles of screening, including sensitivity and specificity of screening tests;
- To be able to carry out pure-tone hearing screening, including the procedures for performing the testing, managing the results, and seeking appropriate follow-up; and
- To be able to carry out immittance-based screening to identify the presence of middle-ear pathology, including screening procedures, management of results, and monitoring necessary follow-up testing.

KEY TERMS AND DEFINITIONS

- **Screening:** A screening program is designed to expediently and reliably identify those likely to have a disorder within the general population. More definitive follow-up testing is typically required to confirm (or refute) the findings of the screening.
- **Test sensitivity:** The proportion of the population or sample who have the disorder or trait for which the screening is being conducted and who failed the screening test (i.e., tested positive for the disorder or trait).
- **Test specificity:** The proportion of the population or sample who do not have the disorder or trait for which the screening is being conducted and who passed the screening test (i.e., tested negative for the disorder or trait).
- **Prevalence:** The estimated proportion of the population who have a particular disorder or trait.

As reviewed in Chapter 5, the audiologist uses a variety of diagnostic tools, including pure-tone audiometry, speech audiometry, and immittance measurements, to determine whether hearing loss or middle-ear dysfunction is present, the severity of the problem, and the likely location of the problem within the auditory system. These results are summarized on audiograms and tympanograms, and are frequently accompanied by a brief written report. For school-aged children with impaired hearing, the speech-language pathologist is often asked to interpret the results obtained by the audiologist so as to incorporate this information into the child's individualized educational plan.

Hearing problems are important to identify at any age. At a young age, the presence of an undetected hearing impairment can have negative consequences for the acquisition and development of speech and language, critical elements of the communication chain. For older adults at the other end of the age continuum, an undetected hearing impairment can impair communication with others and have negative consequences on social and psychological well being.

For many adults, the development of hearing loss is often readily apparent to the hearing-impaired individual and assistance will most likely be sought. This is often not the case, however, for older adults with mild or moderate amounts of sloping, high-frequency, sensorineural hearing loss. Such individuals often wait as long as 10 to 15 years from their (or their spouse's) first suspicion of hearing problems to their first appointment with an audiologist for a complete hearing evaluation. Although it is unclear exactly why this is the case, it has generally been attributed to the negative stigma associated with the use of hearing aids, including the association of hearing-aid use with "old age." The physically invisible inner ear damage accompanying age-related sensorineural hearing loss is suddenly made readily visible to others via the use of a hearing aid or other assistive device. Due to their reluctance to seek assistance, brief, efficient hearing-screening procedures have been developed that can be administered to large numbers of older adults in an effort to identify hearing loss among this population. Once identified, solutions for the hearing loss can be explored and any breaks in the communication chain repaired.

It is very common for hearing loss, and the consequent breaks in the communication chain, to go undetected in children. The younger the child, the more likely this will be the case. Obviously, a newborn or young infant has no way to express that he or she is experiencing difficulty with hearing; they have yet to develop a communication system that would enable them to do so. Even older children, however, with developed communication systems may not realize that a hearing problem they are experiencing, especially one unaccompanied by any physical pain or discomfort, is not "normal" or "typical." For children, we rely heavily on observant parents or caregivers to identify those with

TABLE 6.1	Referral Guidelines for Children with Speech Delay

12 Months
No differentiated babbling or vocal imitation

18 Months
No use of single words

24 Months
Single-word vocabulary ≤10 words

30 Months
Fewer than 100 words, no evidence of two-word combinations, unintelligible

36 Months
Fewer than 200 words, no use of telegraphic sentences, clarity <50%

48 Months
Fewer than 600 words, no use of simple sentences, clarity <80%

From Matkin ND. Early recognition and referral of hearing-impaired children. *Pediatr Rev.* 1984;6:151–156, with permission.

hearing problems. Such problems, however, are often physically invisible to the caregiver, especially for sensorineural hearing loss.

As was noted in Chapter 1, there are typical developmental milestones during the first 4 years of life for speech and language. One way parents or caregivers can identify a possible hearing problem is through observable delays in speech or language development. Table 6.1 provides some guidelines for referral of the child to a professional for a comprehensive assessment, including a hearing evaluation. If a child meets any of these referral guidelines, the parent or caregiver should seek a comprehensive assessment of speech and language capabilities and the child's hearing. Meeting any one of these referral guidelines in Table 6.1 does not mean, however, that the child has hearing loss. Hearing loss is just one of the possible causes of a delay in speech and language development. It is important, however, to rule out hearing loss as the causative factor in the initial assessment.

The referral guidelines in Table 6.1 require observant parents or caregivers, including pediatricians, and assume that the parents and caregivers are familiar with these general guidelines. Note also that these guidelines begin at 12 months of age and several pertain to children 2 years of age or older. As noted in Chapter 1, it would be advantageous to identify hearing problems earlier, before they begin to have a negative impact on the development of speech and language.

How does one go about detecting the presence of significant hearing loss in newborns or young children? One strategy would be to test the hearing and middle-ear function of every newborn and school-aged child. Although it has been estimated that there are 4,000 to 5,000 children born each year in the U.S. with significant hearing loss, this represents only 1 to 3 newborns out of every 1,000 live births. Clearly, it would be extremely costly and inefficient to do complete audiological evaluations on every newborn or every school-aged child. What is needed instead is a simple, efficient, inexpensive way to screen newborns and young children and identify those who are *likely* to have a significant hearing loss. This represents the basic purpose of hearing screening programs for any age group: identify those individuals at risk for hearing loss so that those individuals can have more thorough and comprehensive audiological evaluations to confirm (or refute) the presence of a hearing loss. Again, once such cases have been identified and confirmed through follow-up testing, efforts can then be made to repair the break in the communication chain.

Screening is designed to separate persons who are likely to have an auditory disorder from those who are unlikely to have an auditory disorder and to do so in a simple, safe, rapid, and cost-effective manner. Screening programs are intended to be preventive measures that focus on early identification and subsequent intervention. The objective is to minimize the consequences of hearing loss or middle ear disease as early as possible so that the disorder will not produce a disabling condition.

The purpose of this chapter is to present information on screening for hearing loss and middle ear disease. The review will cover the general principles of screening, discuss screening procedures for hearing loss and otitis media used with different age groups, and recommend follow-up protocols for those identified as having an auditory disorder. The focus in this section is on the screening of children from birth through 18 years of age.

UNDERSTANDING THE PRINCIPLES OF SCREENING

Factors That Determine Whether to Screen

How does one know whether to screen for the presence of a particular disorder? Several criteria are used in establishing the value of screening for a specific disorder. First, a disorder should be important. If left unidentified, the disorder will likely diminish an individual's functional status. It is also essential that the program be capable of reaching those who could benefit. Another important criterion is the prevalence of the disorder, or how frequently it occurs within a given population. There should be acceptable criteria for diagnosis. Specific symptoms of a disease must occur with sufficient regularity that it can be determined with assurance which persons have the disorder and which do not. Once detected, the disease should be treatable. Diagnostic and treatment resources must also be available so that adequate medical and educational follow-up can be implemented. Finally, the health system must be able to cope with the program and the program must be cost effective. It is generally believed by most, but not all, that hearing loss in people of all ages and middle ear disease in children satisfy many of these criteria and that screening for auditory disorders is justifiable.

What Is an Acceptable Screening Test?

A screening test must be selected that will most effectively detect the conditions to be identified. A good screening tool should be acceptable, reliable, valid, safe, and cost effective. An acceptable test is simple, easy to administer, readily interpretable, and generally well received by the public. A reliable test should be consistent, providing results that do not differ significantly from one test to the next for the same individual. It does little good, for example, to have a screening test that the same healthy individual passes five times and fails five times when the test is administered 10 times in succession. Furthermore, the test should allow examiners to be consistent in the evaluation of a response. Two different examiners testing the same person should obtain the same results.

Validity may best be defined by asking, "Are we measuring what we think we are measuring?" The emphasis in this question is on what is being measured. For example, a clinician who wants to identify middle ear disease has selected a screening test that involves the measurement of hearing by air conduction. Such a test would not be valid because, although it might reliably measure a child's hearing loss, it cannot indicate the presence or absence of otitis media. (Recall from the last chapter that a child with a fluid-filled middle ear from otitis media may not have air-conduction thresholds outside the normal range, even though a significant air-bone gap might exist.) Validity of screening tests consists of two components: **sensitivity** and **specificity**. Sensitivity refers to the ability of a screening test to identify accurately an ear that is abnormal (whether from hearing loss or from otitis media); specificity denotes the ability of a screening tool to identify normal ears. Thus, a valid test is one that identifies a normal condition as normal (high specificity) and an abnormal one as abnormal (high sensitivity).

Finally, a good screening test is one that is safe and cost effective in relation to the expected benefits. Because the instruments designed to screen for hearing loss and middle ear disease are considered safe and reasonable in cost, the greatest direct expense is usually the salary for personnel. Other factors should be taken into consideration when estimating the expense of a screening program. These include the time required to administer the test, the cost of supplies, the number of individuals to be screened and rescreened, and the cost of training and supervising screeners.

Calculation of the costs of any screening program should also consider indirect costs, such as the cost of the comprehensive audiologic assessment, monitoring, and intervention that would occur as a result of the screening. A special concern is the cost associated with false-positive tests—those individuals who fail the screen but who have normal hearing. For children, such costs might include a parent's lost time from work, transportation to health care facilities, administration of unnecessary follow-up tests, and, possibly, unnecessary treatment, as well as the more human cost of the anxiety of parents or caring others, the potential of misunderstanding, and the disturbance of family function. Finally, the possible cost savings resulting from a screening program must be entered into the equation. For example, educational costs might be reduced as a consequence of early identification and subsequent intervention.

PRINCIPLES OF EVALUATING A SCREENING TEST

In this section, we will cover some of the basic principles of how to assess the usefulness of a screening test. Figure 6.1 sets the stage for understanding this process. Our primary goal is to distinguish within the population at large those individuals who exhibit an auditory disorder ($A + C$) from those who do not ($B + D$). Within the group with an auditory disorder, subgroup A are those people with the disorder who test positive (true positives); subgroup C are those with the disorder who test negative (false negatives). Within the group without an auditory disorder, subgroup B represents those persons without the disorder who test positive (false positives); subgroup D is comprised of all those persons without the disorder who test negative (true negatives).

Any screening test must be evaluated against an independent standard, often referred to as a "gold standard." The results of the gold standard test are universally accepted as proof that the disease or disorder is either present or absent. In the case of hearing loss, pure-tone audiometry typically serves as the gold standard for any screening tool, whereas for middle ear disease, the gold standard is usually pneumatic otoscopy or electroacoustic immittance.

Figure 6.2 illustrates how the characteristics of a screening test can be evaluated against the gold standard. Toward this end, several terms and definitions need to be understood. The first is sensitivity: $100A/(A + C)$. (The factor 100 is introduced to convert the result to a percentage.) We have already learned

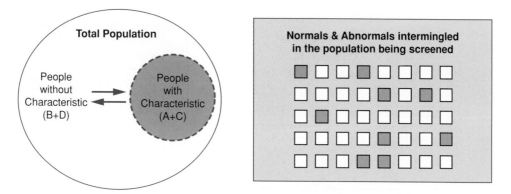

FIGURE 6.1 Illustration of the general notion of screening. On the left, a Venn diagram is used to illustrate that the individuals with a particular disorder represent a subset of the general population and the key is to be able to reliably identify this subset of the population. This is also illustrated on the right where the total set of squares, blue and white, represents the general population; those with the disorder represented by the blue squares and those without the disorder represented by the white squares.

that sensitivity refers to the proportion of individuals with the characteristic correctly identified by the test. If 100 subjects have a hearing loss and the test correctly identifies 75 of them, the sensitivity of the test would be 75%. In Figure 6.2, the sensitivity is $100(7/9)$, or 77.8%. Sensitivity is typically affected by the severity or duration of the characteristic or disease. This is only logical in that the milder an impairment is, the closer it is to a normal condition and the more difficult it is to distinguish from normal. However, the measure is not affected by how prevalent the disease is in the general population.

Another important measure is specificity: $100D/(B + D)$. Specificity refers to the proportion of individuals without the characteristic correctly identified by the test. If in a group of 100 normal subjects, the test identifies 70 as normal and 30 as abnormal, the specificity would be 70%. In Figure 6.2, the specificity is $100(27/31)$, or 87.1%. Like sensitivity, specificity is not affected by the prevalence of the disorder. The best screening tool will be one that provides the highest degree of both sensitivity and specificity.

It is possible to vary the accuracy of a screening test by altering the pass/fail criteria. A cutoff on a hearing screening test, for example, might be 15 dB HL or 40 dB HL. A 15-dB HL cutoff will provide high sensitivity but lower specificity. This is because the 15-dB HL criterion will result in a larger portion of near-normal subjects being classified as hearing-impaired. If a 40-dB HL cutoff is used, however, sensitivity will decrease but specificity will increase. The 40-dB HL cutoff will miss some of the mildly impaired near-normal subjects but will avoid misclassifying most of the subjects with normal hearing.

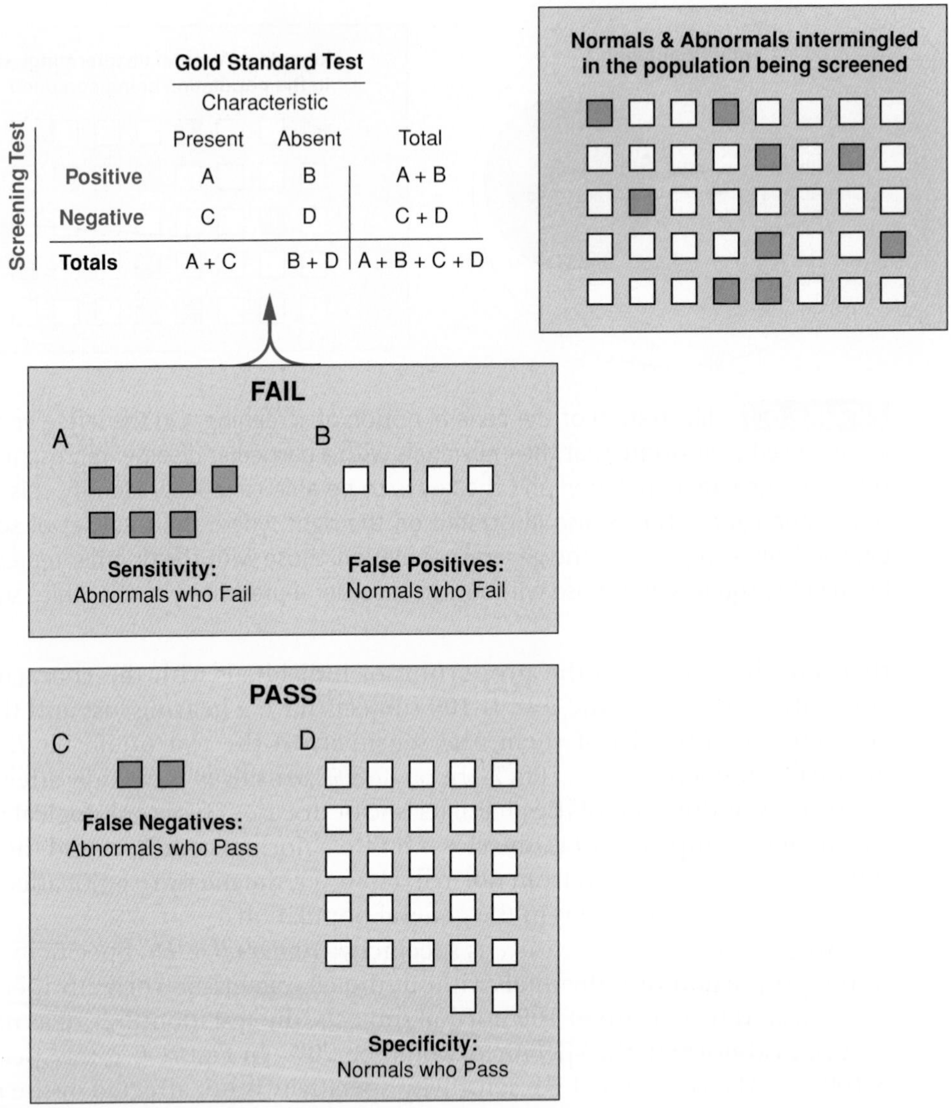

FIGURE 6.2 Schematic illustration of the "sorting" of the general population (all squares) into those who have the disorder ("fail") and those who do not ("pass"), according to the screening test used, compared to their true grouping (blue or white squares). Ideally, the individuals represented by blue squares, those who truly have the disorder, would be the only ones who fail the screening and those represented by the white squares, who do not have the disorder, would be the only ones who pass. Errors of both types, passing those who have the disorder (group C) and failing those who do not (group B), are almost always made. The table at the left illustrates the four subgroups, A through D, in tabular format, together with various column and row sums used in the evaluation of a screening test.

An important concept in any screening program is the prevalence of the disorder that is to be screened. **Prevalence** (derived from the word *prevail*) refers to the proportion of individuals in the population who demonstrate the characteristic $[100(A + C)/(A + B + C + D)]$. An important use of prevalence data is as a pretest indicator of the probability of the disorder being present. To illustrate how the prevalence of a disorder may be important to a screening program, consider the following two extremes. If 99% of the population has the disorder, it is easier to simply assume that everyone has it and treat it accordingly. In this case, we would only be mistreating 1% of the population. If one in a million people have the disorder (prevalence = 0.0001%), then it may be safer and more efficient to assume that no one has it. Failure to screen for such a disorder would miss 0.0001% of the population.

In most hearing clinic settings, especially when screening for hearing loss, we need tests that yield maximum accuracy. The ideal test would be one that always gave positive results in anyone with a hearing loss and negative results in anyone without a hearing loss. Unfortunately, no such test exists. As a rule, one attempts to maximize the sensitivity and specificity of a screening test. This is done by evaluating different pass/fail criteria and test protocols in comparison to the gold standard. Vignettes 6.1 and 6.2 give examples of how to apply these general principles to actual screening data.

STATUS OF IDENTIFICATION PROGRAMS IN THE UNITED STATES

Screening: A Common Healthcare Practice

No single procedure in healthcare is more popular than that of screening. Tests are performed for a variety of conditions including blood pressure, cholesterol, genetics, diabetes, breast cancer, colorectal cancer, other types of cancer, and of course, hearing and middle-ear status. New screening tests are developed each year and legislation is always being introduced to mandate a given screening protocol. It is important to recognize that screening tests usually lead to additional procedures, which in turn constitute a large part of today's healthcare practice. It is one of the factors that contribute to the high costs of healthcare. For example, the billions of dollars expended for just three of the widely recognized screening programs (cervical cancer, prostate cancer, and high blood levels of cholesterol) are sufficient to fund a basic healthcare system for all of the poor and uninsured. Today's healthcare system actively encourages us to obtain screenings for a variety of conditions. Vignette 6.3 highlights a typical screening advertisement published in a local newspaper and illustrates how such screening advertisements can sometimes mislead the consumer.

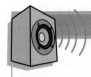

VIGNETTE 6.1   CONCEPTUAL DEMO

GUIDELINES FOR CALCULATING THE OPERATING CHARACTERISTICS OF A SCREENING TOOL

Let us now go through the step-by-step procedures for calculating the characteristics of a screening tool. To assist in this process, some screening data are presented. The gold standard was pure-tone audiometry. In this example, a total of 99 patients were screened and then tested using pure-tone audiometry. It is noted that 47 patients failed the screening test, 27 of whom actually had a hearing impairment and 20 of whom did not. On the other hand, 52 patients passed the screening. Of these, the gold standard showed that three had a hearing loss and 49 did not. The prevalence of hearing loss in the population screened $[100(A + C)/(A + B + C + D)]$ is $100(30/99)$, or approximately 30%.

First, the sensitivity, or the percentage of valid positive test results, is calculated from the data. The formula for computing sensitivity is $100A/(A + C)$. When applied to our data, this gives $100(27/30) = 90\%$. This is excellent.

Next, compute specificity, or the percentage of valid negative test results, using the formula $100D/(B + D)$. This results in $100(49/69) = 71\%$. This is adequate but not excellent.

In this example, we see that the screening test seems to be a valid tool for the identification of a hearing loss, offering acceptable sensitivity and specificity values. Now, on your own, calculate the operating characteristics of a screening tool for the example in Vignette 6.2.

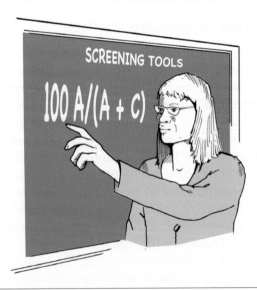

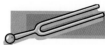

VIGNETTE 6.2   EXPERIMENT

COMPUTING THE CHARACTERISTICS OF A SCREENING TOOL USING HYPOTHETICAL SCREENING DATA

Now compute the characteristics of a screening tool for the example shown below. For this example, compute prevalence, sensitivity, and specificity.

Example:

GOLD STANDARD TEST

	Hearing Impairment Characteristic		
Screening Test	Present	Absent	Total
Fail	160	20	180
Pass	40	180	220
Total	200	200	400

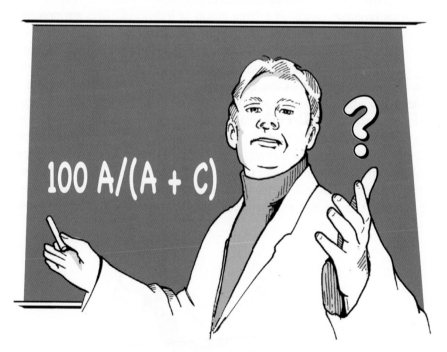

How did you do? You can find the answers in the back of the chapter.

VIGNETTE 6.3 FURTHER DISCUSSION

SCREENING IS A POPULAR PROCEDURE IN TODAY'S HEALTHCARE ENVIRONMENT

Screening is one of the most popular procedures in healthcare, and healthcare facilities aggressively promote the need to be screened for a variety of conditions. The figure below illustrates a typical advertisement seen in a local community newspaper. The advertisement states "one out of every 11 men will develop prostate cancer with the risk rising dramatically after the age of 40." The message is clear, the risk is high, and we better get screened for this condition right away. Unfortunately, the information presented in this advertisement does not tell the whole story. The digital rectal examination used for screening prostate cancer is not a very accurate test. Studies illustrate that when we screen asymptomatic males, the examination will only detect approximately 33% of those with cancer; the test misses the vast majority of cases. Moreover, the test produces many false positives. Less than one-third of the positive tests actually turn out to be cancer, whereas two-thirds or more of the failures will be false-positives. This means that the test suggests probable cancer in a large group of individuals who are normal. Hence, many individuals who fail the test but do not have cancer will be referred for additional tests, thus adding to the costs of the screening program, not to mention the cost of fear, anxiety, confusion, and misunderstanding. Finally, it is important to point out that there is no evidence to suggest that the digital rectal screening is worthwhile. No one has shown that individuals who are screened for this problem are any better off than those who are not screened. This lack of evidence has caused some national groups to recommend against this type of screening for prostate cancer. The lesson is that just because a screening procedure is popular and we are encouraged to be screened by healthcare facilities, this does not necessarily mean the screening is beneficial. To determine whether a screening procedure is beneficial, we must first consider the principles of screening discussed earlier in this chapter and then apply these principles to the available evidence.

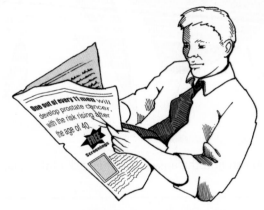

Hearing and Immittance Screening Programs for Children

Identification programs for hearing loss in children have been implemented in the United States for various age groups including the neonate, the infant, the preschooler, and the school-aged child. Despite the importance of early identification, most screening has occurred at the school-aged level. It has only been within the past 5 to 7 years that newborn hearing screening has become widespread; in fact, because of the undaunted efforts of Marion Downs (see Vignette 6.4) and others, more than 40 states now mandate universal newborn screening.

Interestingly, many pediatricians do not recognize the importance of screening very young infants for hearing loss. It has been estimated, for example, that only 3% of children from 6 months to 11 years of age receive a screening test at their primary health-care source. Although it is true that more reliable responses can be obtained from infants and young children than from neonates, there is the problem of locating all of the older groups of youngsters for the hearing test. Once newborns leave the hospital, it is not until age 5 years, at the kindergarten level, that these children are available for testing at one common location. Those few screening programs that do exist are conducted in day-care centers, well-baby clinics, and head-start programs. These programs, however, attract only a specific segment of children. Even if a massive national effort were made to screen all preschoolers at these various centers, a large percentage of children would still be missed. Yet screening the preschool child has some advantages over the screening of newborns. First, children become easier to test as age increases and yield more reliable and valid results. Second, children with progressive hearing loss and those whose hearing loss was not detected at the newborn screening stand a good chance of being identified.

Under our present system, children whose hearing loss was not detected at the newborn identification program or who moved into a community at preschool age are not identified until screening occurs in kindergarten. There is a critical need for a national effort directed at infant and preschool hearing screening programs in every state.

Hearing screening programs using pure-tone audiometry are most often conducted in the school system because it affords easy access to the children. However, the availability, accessibility, comprehensiveness, and quality of school screening programs vary significantly from one state to the next. A major problem and source of frustration for audiologists involved in school screening programs is the lack of appropriate follow-up services offered to children who fail the screen.

The incorporation of immittance screening programs is not as universal. It is estimated that about one half of the states incorporate immittance

VIGNETTE 6.4 HISTORICAL NOTE

MARION P. DOWNS, (1914–) "ADVOCATE FOR EARLY IDENTIFICATION FOR HEARING LOSS IN INFANTS"

Throughout her professional career, Marion Downs championed the early identification of hearing loss in very young infants. Recognizing the value of early auditory stimulation while teaching at the University of Denver in the early 1950's, she introduced the concept of early identification. After entering the faculty of the University of Colorado Medical School in 1959 she was able to implement the concept by developing a comprehensive early identification program for all newborns in the Denver area and screened more than 10,000 babies using the "arousal test." This test was later judged to be impractical. Consequently, Downs proposed to the American Speech-Language-Hearing Association the formation of the National Joint Committee on Infant Hearing and chaired the committee in its first few years. The committee continues to be instrumental in promoting the concept of Universal Newborn Hearing Screening. Downs served as an advocate for early identification and habilitation throughout the world as a consultant to foreign governments and by presenting workshops and lectures in some 18 different countries. In 1997, Ms. Downs was honored by having a national center on hearing and infants named after her. The center promotes her lifelong dream of achieving early intervention for newborns not only in Colorado but throughout the country. Now in retirement, Downs continues to advance her long ideal of newborn hearing screening and early intervention. In October, 2007, Downs received the Secretary's Highest Recognition Award from the U.S. Department of Health and Human Services for her work in the areas of early identification and intervention.

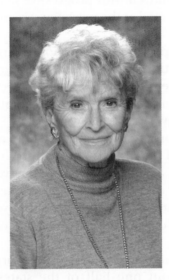

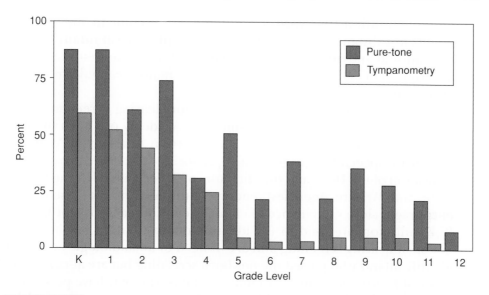

FIGURE 6.3 Percent of school-age children receiving either air-conduction pure-tone hearing screening or tympanometric screening as a function of grade level. (Tympanometry data from Roush J. Screening school-age children. In Bess FH, Hall JW, eds. *Screening Children for Auditory Function.* Nashville: Bill Wilkerson Center Press; 1992; Pure-tone data from Penn. T: A summary: School-based hearing screening in the United States. *Andiology Today*, 11, 20–21, 1999.)

(tympanometry) as part of their screening procedures. Some of the problems associated with mass immittance screening are discussed later in this chapter.

Figure 6.3 shows the percentage of school programs that conduct pure-tone and immittance screening. It is seen that the emphasis for pure-tone and immittance screening in the schools is at the elementary level and that few programs conduct screening in the secondary grades. Moreover, a much larger percentage of school programs use pure-tone screening than immittance screening.

Screening the Neonate

The advantages of detecting sensorineural hearing loss as early as possible in young children are important enough to encourage the implementation of newborn screening programs. It has now been demonstrated that children who receive intervention from the age of 3 years or younger show significantly better speech and language outcomes later in life. Early identification and intervention (the word *intervene* means "to come in and modify") also results in substantial cost savings. For example, a Deaf infant who receives educational and audiologic management during the first years of life has a better than 50% chance of becoming "mainstreamed" into a regular classroom.

The National Joint Committee on Infant Hearing Screening (a committee of representatives from the American Academy of Otolaryngology, the American Academy of Pediatrics, the American Academy of Audiology, the American Speech-Language-Hearing Association (ASHA), the Council on Education of the Deaf, and the Directors of Speech and Hearing Programs in State and Welfare Agencies) endorses universal newborn screening and encourages close surveillance of children considered at-risk for hearing loss. Risk indicators are used to (1) identify infants who did not have access to newborn hearing screening and are in need of an audiologic evaluation; (2) identify infants who passed the newborn screening but are at-risk for delayed onset of hearing loss; and (3) identify infants who may have passed the newborn screening but have mild forms of permanent sensorineural hearing loss. Table 6.2 lists the 2007 Joint Committee's risk indicators. Infants who possess any one of these risk indicators should receive periodic audiologic monitoring, medical surveillance, and ongoing observation of communication development. Those children with risk indicators that are associated with delayed-onset hearing loss should receive heightened audiologic and medical surveillance.

Auditory Brainstem Response

The auditory brainstem response (ABR; Chapter 3) has been suggested as a reliable indicator of hearing sensitivity in infancy. The advantages of the ABR for newborn screening include: (a) the use of less intense, near-threshold stimuli, making it possible to detect milder forms of hearing impairment; (b) the ability to detect both unilateral and bilateral hearing losses; and (c) the use of a physiologic measurement that depends entirely on a sensory response. Limitations to the technique include the cost and sophisticated nature of the instrumentation, the use of an acoustic click that makes the ABR primarily sensitive to only high-frequency hearing loss, and the fact that the ABR is not a conscious response at the level of the cortex (presence of an ABR does not mean the individual can hear). Nevertheless, the measure is thought to provide a good estimate of hearing status when used carefully, especially when one considers the limitations of the alternative procedures. A child who fails an ABR screening in the intensive-care nursery must be retested later under more favorable conditions.

TABLE 6.2 **Risk Indicators Associated with Permanent Congenital, Delayed-Onset, or Progressive Hearing Loss in Childhood**

Risk indicators in blue font are of greater concern for delayed-onset hearing loss.

1. Caregiver concern regarding hearing, speech, language, or developmental delay.
2. Family history of permanent childhood hearing loss.
3. Neonatal intensive care of more than 5 days or any of the following regardless of length of stay: ECMO, assisted ventilation, exposure to ototoxic medications (gentimycin and tobramycin) or loop diuretics (furosemide/Lasix), and hyperbilirubinemia that requires exchange transfusion.
4. In utero infections, such as CMV, herpes, rubella, syphilis, and toxoplasmosis.
5. Craniofacial anomalies, including those that involve the pinna, ear canal, ear tags, ear pits, and temporal bone anomalies.
6. Physical findings, such as white forelock, that are associated with a syndrome known to include a sensorineural or permanent conductive hearing loss.
7. Syndromes associated with hearing loss or progressive or late-onset hearing loss, such as neurofibromatosis, osteopetrosis, and Usher syndrome; other frequently identified syndromes include Waardenburg, Alport, Pendred, and Jervell and Lange-Nielson.
8. Neurodegenerative disorders, such as Hunter syndrome, or sensory motor neuropathies, such as Friedreich ataxia and Charcot-Marie-Tooth syndrome.
9. Culture-positive postnatal infections associated with sensorineural hearing loss, including confirmed bacterial and viral (especially herpes viruses and varicella) meningitis.
10. Head trauma, especially basal skull/temporal bone fracture that requires hospitalization.
11. Chemotherapy.

Adapted from Joint Committee on Infant Hearing. Year 2007 Position Statement: Principles and Guidelines for Early Hearing Detection and Intervention Programs. *Pediatrics*. 2007; 120:898-921.

Several ABR-based screening systems with automated response collection and evaluation have been designed for use with neonates. These devices are portable, automatic, and microprocessor-based. Their primary function is to screen for handicapping hearing loss in newborn infants. These simplified and cost-effective systems use various automated algorithms to determine whether an infant passes or fails. These devices are generally preferred for screening because they do not require test interpretation, they reduce the possible influence of tester bias, and they insure test consistency.

Otoacoustic Emissions

As noted in Chapter 3, evoked otoacoustic emissions (OAEs) have been used as a screening tool to identify hearing loss in neonates. Although there is some disagreement as to the details of such a screening protocol, including which type of OAE to use and the appropriate stimulus parameters to optimize screening efficiency, the scientific and clinical communities have recommended that OAEs become an integral part of a universal neonatal hearing screening program for the United States. It has generally been recommended that either OAEs or ABR be used for the initial screening, with all screening failures retested with the alternative measure. Many of the advantages and disadvantages described for the use of ABR as a screening tool also apply to the use of OAEs as a screening measure. One limitation to OAE is that the test will not identify individuals with neural complications.

Screening the Infant and Preschool-Aged Child
Identification Tests and Procedures

Selection of screening techniques will depend on the age, maturity, and cooperation of the child. Generally speaking, a test using sound localization in the sound field will be required for those children between the ages of 4 months and 2 years. Conventional audiometric screening using earphones can usually be used with children 3 years of age or older. Children between the ages of 2 and 3 years make up the most difficult group for which to select an appropriate test. Some of these children can be conditioned for traditional screening techniques with earphones, whereas others will require the test based on sound localization.

Infant and Pre-Nursery Child (4 Months to 3 Years)

Certainly, OAEs or ABR may be used to screen this population for hearing loss. Too often, however, these devices are not available in settings where infants and preschool age children are typically screened.

The use of calibrated acoustic stimuli (e.g., narrow-band noise) is often suggested for eliciting a localization (head turn) response in a sound field setting. The child is placed on the parent's lap and the acoustic stimulus is presented about 2 feet from either ear. If the child fails to localize the signal, a rescreening is recommended. A second failure results in a third test 1 week later. If the child again fails the test, a complete diagnostic examination is conducted. Unfortunately, this technique does not offer ear-specific information and a child with unilateral hearing loss will probably be missed.

Sometimes, delays in speech/language development are the most sensitive and valid indicators of hearing impairment among preschool children. It has been suggested that primary-care physicians and other allied health personnel screen young children for hearing loss simply by asking the parent three basic questions: (a) How many different words do you estimate your child uses? Is it 100 words, 500 words, etc.?; (b) What is the length of a typical sentence that your child uses? Is it single words, two words, full sentences, etc.?; and (c) How clear is your child's speech to a friend or neighbor? Would they understand 10%, 50%, 90%, etc.? These questions are framed around the referral guidelines shown previously in Table 6.1.

#21

Preschooler (3 to 6 Years)

When the child reaches 3 years of age, the more traditional hearing test with earphones can be used for screening. By means of a portable pure-tone audiometer, signals may be presented at various frequencies at a fixed intensity level. The child merely indicates to the examiner, usually by raising a hand, if a tone was perceived. The ASHA has recommended that 1,000, 2,000, and 4,000 Hz be used as test frequencies. If immittance testing is not part of the program, the frequency 500 Hz should also be tested (assuming that background noise levels in the test area are acceptable). The ASHA further recommends a screening level of 20 dB HL for all frequencies tested. A lack of response at any frequency in either ear constitutes a test failure. Children who fail should be rescreened, preferably within the same test session, but no later than 1 week after the original test. The practice of rescreening can significantly reduce the overall number of test failures. The value of rescreening is illustrated in Figure 6.4, which shows that the total number of

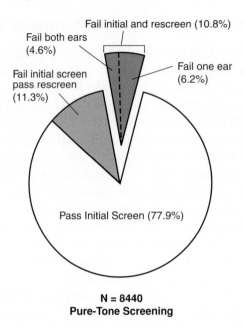

Fail initial and rescreen (10.8%)

Fail both ears (4.6%)

Fail initial screen pass rescreen (11.3%)

Fail one ear (6.2%)

Pass Initial Screen (77.9%)

N = 8440
Pure-Tone Screening

FIGURE 6.4 ▪ Illustration of importance of re-screening. Originally, 22.1% (11.3% + 10.8%) failed initial screening, but only about half of those (10.8%) failed both screenings. (Adapted from Wilson WR, Walton WK. Public School Audiometry. In Martin, FN, ed. *Pediatric Audiology*. Englewood Cliffs, NJ: Prentice-Hall, 1978.)

failures has been significantly reduced via rescreening. Children who also fail the rescreening should be referred for a complete audiologic evaluation.

Procedural Considerations for Preschool-Aged Children   In developing a screening program at the preschool level, special attention should be directed toward the groundwork and orientation process that occurs before the screening. The success of any screening program depends, to a large extent, on the cooperation of the teachers, the children, and the parents. All three of these parties must be familiarized with the screening process that is to take place.

First, a letter should go to the teacher outlining the need for and the purpose of the screening program. The letter should also review the teacher's responsibilities in preparing the children for the screening. Prescreening instructional activities can be used by the teacher to orient the children to the listening task. Such activities performed before the identification program can help avoid wasted time during the actual screening. It is also most helpful to provide the teacher with a list of the screening responsibilities of those individuals who will be conducting the screening, as well as of those who will be receiving the screening. This list will serve as an excellent guide and provide the teacher and/or administrator with a better understanding of the entire screening process from start to finish. Finally, a sample letter to the parents of each child should be included in the packet of materials, as well as a parental consent form. The letter should explain the screening program so that the parents will understand the value of screening and support the screening process.

The person who will be responsible for conducting the screening program should visit the facility and meet with the teacher(s) and administrator(s). Together they should review carefully the sequence of the screening program and discuss any concerns they might have. This is also an excellent opportunity to review with the program officials the sites available for the screening. Needless to say, a quiet room is essential. Other considerations in selecting a testing site have been identified by others. The site should: (a) have appropriate electrical outlets (only grounded three-prong outlets should be used) and lighting; (b) be located away from railroad tracks, playgrounds, heavy traffic, public toilets, or cafeterias; (c) be relatively free of visual distractions; (d) have carpet and curtains to help reduce the room noise; (e) have nearby bathroom facilities to accommodate the needs of the children and screeners; and (f) have chairs and tables appropriate for small children.

Some other suggestions and hints for screening preschool children include the following. One person should be individually responsible for ensuring that the children move through the screening process smoothly and that all children receive the test. Arrangements should be made for the children to have name tags showing their legal names and nicknames. All forms should be accurately completed before the screening date. Each child should have his or her own individual preschool record form. When screening children between the ages of 3 and 6 years, it is wise to alternate age groups during the screening day; for example, 3-year-olds should be followed by 5-year-olds. Three-year olds are much harder to test and take more time. Another factor to keep in mind is that the younger children tire more easily than older children and need to be screened earlier in the day.

Screening the School-Aged Child

The practice of screening school-aged children is over 50 years old, and all states conduct some form of hearing screening in the schools. The Joint Committee on Health Problems in Education (consisting of members of the National Educational Association and the American Medical Association) has described the following primary responsibilities to be met by a screening program: an awareness of the importance of early recognition of suspected hearing loss, especially in the primary grades; intelligent observation of pupils for signs of hearing difficulty; organization and conduction of an audiometric screening survey; and a counseling and follow-up program to help children with hearing difficulties obtain diagnostic examinations, needed treatment, and such adaptations of their school program as their hearing condition dictates.

Who Is Responsible for the Audiometric Screening Program?

Health and education departments are the agents primarily responsible for coordinating audiometric screening programs. Ideally, the state's department of education should coordinate the periodic screening of all school children as well as provide for the necessary educational, audiologic, and rehabilitative follow-up. The state's department of health, on the other hand, should coordinate the activities of identification audiometry, threshold measurement, and medical follow-up for students who fail the screening tests.

Personnel

The personnel designated to conduct the screening tests have been nurses, audiologists, speech-language pathologists, graduate students in speech and hearing, and even volunteers and secretaries. To assure quality programs, only professionals trained in audiology should be used to coordinate and supervise hearing screening programs. Volunteers and lay groups can best be used for support, such as in the promotion of screening programs. Certified audiologists or speech-language pathologists should oversee screening programs and use trained assistants or technicians to perform the screening. Public health nurses may serve as organizers and supervisors but can be of most value in the follow-up phase of the program. A nurse's responsibilities might include: (a) counseling parents and children about the child's needs for medical diagnosis and treatment, (b) using all available facilities for diagnosis and treatment, and (c) coordinating information about the child and family with specialists in the health and education field.

Who Should Be Screened?

It is not economically feasible to mass screen all children in the schools. A target population must be identified. Most programs have concentrated their annual screening efforts on children of nursery-school age through grade 3. In fact, all of these grades are recommended for screening by the ASHA guidelines. After grade 3, children may be screened at 3- to 4-year intervals. By concentrating the screening efforts on the first 3 or 4 years of school, it is still possible to carefully observe other special groups of school children. Several groups of children require more attention than is provided by routine screening. Included among these groups are children with pre-existing hearing loss, multiple handicaps, frequent colds or ear infections, delayed language, or defective speech. In addition, children who are returning to school after a serious illness, enrolled in special education programs, experiencing school failure, exhibiting sudden change in academic performance, referred by the classroom teacher, or new to the school also require more attention to their hearing than provided by routinely scheduled screenings.

Equipment, Calibration, and the Test Environment

An important component of any identification program is the audiometric equipment used in the screening. The equipment needed for individual pure-tone screening should be simple, sturdy, and portable. Most screening audiometers are portable and weigh as little as 2 or 3 pounds. The performance characteristics of these instruments must remain stable over time. An audiometer that does not perform adequately could result in a higher-than-normal false-positive or false-negative rate. Care should be taken to ensure that all of the equipment used in screening satisfies the national performance standards. Unfortunately, this is not always done. Audiometers used in the schools often fail to meet calibration standards. School audiometers should receive weekly intensity checks with a sound level meter, as well as daily listening performance checks. All aspects of the audiometer should be thoroughly calibrated each year. It is also suggested that spare audiometers be available in case a malfunction occurs during a screening identification program.

Older audiometers will be most subject to instability and malfunction and should receive careful surveillance. Clinical audiologists who use these instruments for threshold measurement (after a screen failure) should know that the masking stimuli generated by many of these portable audiometers are often inadequate.

Once again, screening must be conducted in a quiet environment to ensure accurate measurements. Although some modern schools have sound-treated rooms or mobile units with testing facilities, most do not. Screening programs must be conducted in a relatively quiet room designed for some other purpose. Some helpful guidelines for selecting an appropriate room for screening have been outlined in the section on preschool screening.

Screening Procedures

The ASHA guidelines for pure-tone air-conduction hearing screening are the most widely used in the schools. The ASHA procedures recognized that sound-treated environments were not readily available in the schools and focus only on middle and higher frequencies. In particular, screening is conducted at 20 dB HL at 1,000, 2,000, and 4,000 Hz in each ear. Failure to detect any one of these pure tones results in the failure of the screening. It is recommended that all failures be rescreened at a later date prior to referral for a complete audiological evaluation.

Why do these specific values for hearing level (20 dB HL) and these three frequencies (1,000, 2,000, and 4,000 Hz) form the basis of screening guidelines for school-age children by ASHA? As described in Chapter 5, for example, the normal limits for hearing threshold are generally considered to be 0 to 25 dB HL at each frequency. Why not screen at 25 dB HL? Briefly, because of the potential negative impact of even very mild hearing loss on the educational development of children, the maximum amount of hearing loss tolerable in school-aged children is considered to be 20 dB HL instead of 25 dB HL.

What about other test frequencies? Are we not concerned about hearing loss at frequencies of 250 or 500 Hz in addition to that from 1,000 through 4,000 Hz? Yes, we are concerned about hearing loss at all of these frequencies. However, because most test environments in which the screening is conducted have high noise levels at the lower frequencies, it is often not possible to get valid results for pure-tone screening at these lower frequencies. Inclusion of these lower frequencies would result in many more children failing the screening and requiring follow-up testing, but not necessarily due to the presence of hearing loss. Rather, they may fail simply because the background noise at the time of testing was too great at the lower frequencies and made it impossible to hear sounds softer than 20 dB HL, even while wearing earphones. The severity of hearing loss at 1,000 Hz is related in most cases to the severity of hearing loss at 500 Hz. In that sense, inclusion of 1,000 Hz in the screening protocol provides indirect information about the child's hearing status at 500 Hz. (NOTE: Please use the interactive pure-tone hearing screens located on the accompanying CD.)

Finally, it cannot be overemphasized that screening is designed to identify those "at risk" for hearing loss, not to confirm the presence of hearing loss. Thus, failure of the hearing screening does not mean that the person has hearing loss. It simply means that the child "probably has" or "may have" hearing loss. Only through a complete follow-up audiological evaluation can the presence of hearing loss be confirmed.

IDENTIFICATION OF MIDDLE EAR DISEASE IN CHILDREN

Electroacoustic Immittance

There is considerable interest in using electroacoustic immittance measures to identify middle ear disease among children. Several factors have contributed to the interest in using immittance as a screening tool. Some factors relate to immittance in particular, and others relate to screening for middle ear disease in general. These factors include the ease and rapidity with which immittance measurement can obtain accurate information, the relative ineffectiveness of pure-tone audiometry in detecting a middle ear disorder, the high prevalence of otitis media, and the growing awareness of the medical, psychological, and educational consequences that may result from middle ear disease. Today this popular technique is used routinely, not only in audiology centers but also in public health facilities, pediatricians' and otologists' offices, and schools.

A problem with immittance screening has been the difficulty of developing appropriate pass/fail criteria. The pass/fail criteria developed have often resulted in unacceptably high referral rates (32% to 36%). The screening criteria known as the Hirtshal program seem to produce a better result. The program uses only tympanometry and does not include the acoustic reflex. At the first screen, all children with normal tympanograms are cleared. The remaining children receive a second screen in 4 to 6 weeks, and all cases with flat tympanograms are referred. Those children still remaining receive a third screen 4 to 6 weeks later. Children with normal tympanograms or tympanograms having peaks in the range of -100 to -199 daPa are cleared. Children with flat tympanograms (and equivalent ear-canal volume outside the normal range) or tympanograms with peaks ≤-200 daPa at the third screen are referred. With the Hirtshal screening approach, sensitivity and specificity values are 80% and 95%, respectively. Moreover, the program yields an acceptable referral rate of only 9%.

The ASHA developed a new guideline for screening children that involves the use of case history, visual inspection of the ear canal and eardrum, and tympanometry with a low frequency (220 or 226 Hz) probe tone. The ASHA recommended that children be screened as needed or if an at-risk condition existed. Children 7 months to 6 years of age should be screened if they present with any of the following conditions: (a) first episode of acute otitis media before 6 months of age; (b) were bottle-fed; (c) have craniofacial anomalies, stigmata, or other syndromic conditions; (d) are members of ethnic populations known to have a higher prevalence of middle ear disease (Native Americans and Eskimo populations); (e) have a family history of middle ear disease with effusion; (f) reside in daycare or in crowded conditions; (g) have been exposed frequently to cigarette smoke; or (h) have been diagnosed with sensorineural hearing loss, learning disabilities, or other developmental complications.

Typically, the first scheduled screening program should occur in the fall in conjunction with screening for hearing loss. A second scheduled screening is recommended for those who failed or were missed in the fall.

For case history, the protocol simply considers recent evidence of otalgia (earache) or otorrhea (discharge from the ear). Visual inspection via otoscopy is performed to identify gross abnormalities; the use of a lighted otoscope or video-otoscope is recommended. A child is referred for medical observation and/or audiologic evaluation if: (a) ear drainage is observed; (b) structural defects or ear canal abnormalities are seen in the ear; (c) tympanometry reveals a flat tympanogram and equivalent ear-canal volume outside normal range; and (d) tympanometric rescreen results are outside test criteria. It should be noted that data pertaining to the performance of this protocol are limited.

Handheld Tympanometers

Small portable handheld immittance screening tympanometers are often used in screening programs. These handheld otoscope-like units typically run on rechargeable batteries and incorporate a small printer to record a hard copy of the data. The tip of the tympanometer is placed into the ear, and when a pneumatic seal is obtained, a microcomputer initiates the miniature pump that varies pressure to the ear canal from +200 daPa to −300 daPa with a 226-Hz probe tone at 85 dB SPL. These handheld screening instruments record data recommended by the ASHA Immittance Screening Guidelines.

FOLLOW-UP

Screening is of little value if follow-up is not provided for the appropriate management of children who fail the screen. This aspect of the program takes as much planning and effort as any other phase of the screening program. Noncompliance has been one of the principal problems of existing hearing screening programs for newborns. In some studies, 25% to 80% of infants who failed newborn screening have been lost to follow-up despite aggressive recruiting efforts and the offering of cost-saving incentives to parents. In other studies, after early identification of hearing loss, lag times of 8 to 9 months have transpired before infants returned for intervention services. Presently, there are no data on compliance in hearing screening programs for infants beyond the newborn period.

For preschool and school-aged programs, the screening coordinator will be responsible for the follow-up under most circumstances. A child who fails the rescreen should receive a comprehensive audiologic test at the screening site as soon as possible. Within a few days after the screening, those steps essential to appropriate follow-up should begin. Letters should be sent to parents indicating whether their child passed or failed the screening test. For those children who failed the screening, the letter should also recommend that the child be referred for medical evaluation. Approximately 6 weeks after the screening, the parents should be asked whether the recommendations were followed.

Frequently, the public health nurse handles this phase of the follow-up program. In some states, audiologists, speech-language pathologists, and educators coordinate this activity. After the medical examination, the child is referred to an audiologic facility for comprehensive testing and counseling. Parent counseling is an important aspect of the follow-up process and too often is overlooked by the supervisors of screening programs. Parents must receive special assistance and guidance to understand and cope with the prospect of having a hearing-impaired child. They must receive help before they can help their child.

Finally, the child will need to be referred to educational services that will be used for planning and placement. The follow-up is a lengthy and ongoing process requiring close coordination among all persons involved.

SUMMARY

Often it is more important to efficiently determine in a large group of children if there are breaks in any child's communication chain, rather then pinpointing the exact nature and severity of the break. Screening programs have been designed and developed for just this purpose. We have defined and justified screening and discussed important considerations and techniques of identification programs. Identification is an important first step in the overall hearing conservation program. The early identification of hearing loss and middle ear disease is the key to effective and appropriate management. There is still much to be learned about our screening programs for the identification of both hearing loss and middle ear disease. In particular, we need to learn more about the feasibility of universal screening of healthy newborns. Other critical issues, such as performance of screening tools, accessibility and availability of follow-up services, compliance, and costs, need to be further explored. There is also a need for more research on screening with immittance for middle ear disease in children.

CHAPTER REVIEW QUESTIONS

1. What is the basic purpose of any screening program?
2. What are some of the desirable features of screening tests?
3. What do sensitivity and specificity of a screening test indicate? What are ideal values for each? What are typical values for screening for hearing loss in newborns?
4. If 1 in 100 million Americans suffered from a serious life-threatening disease, would it be appropriate to screen all Americans for this disorder? Why or why not? What other factors might need to be considered?
5. If 99.9 million of every 100 million Americans suffered from a serious disease, would it be appropriate to screen all Americans for this disorder? Why or why not? What other factors might need to be considered?

SUGGESTED READINGS

American Academy of Pediatrics. Newborn and infant hearing loss: Detection and intervention. Taskforce on Newborn and Infant Hearing. *Pediatrics.* 1999;103:527–530.

American National Standards Institute. *American National Standards Specifications for Audiometers.* ANSI S3.6-1989. New York: American National Standards Institute; 1989.

American Speech-Language-Hearing Association. *Guidelines for Audiologic Screening.* Rockville, MD: ASHA Desk Reference, 1997.

American Speech-Language-Hearing Association. Considerations in screening adults/older persons for handicapping hearing impairments. *ASHA.* 1992; 34:81–87.

Bess FH. *Children With Hearing Impairment: Contemporary Trends.* Nashville: Vanderbilt Bill Wilkerson Center Press; 1998.

Bess FH, Gravel JS. *Foundations of Pediatric Audiology: A Book of Readings.* San Diego, CA: Plural Publishing; 2006.

Bess FH, Hall JW. *Screening Children for Auditory Function.* Nashville: Bill Wilkerson Center Press; 1992.

Bess FH, Penn TO. Issues and concerns associated with universal newborn hearing screening programs. *J Speech-Lang Pathol Audiol.* 2001;24:113–123.

Downs M. Early identification of hearing loss: Where are we? Where do we go from here? In: Mencher GT, ed. *Early Identification of Hearing Loss.* Basel, Switzerland: S Karger; 1976.

Harford ER, Bess FH, Bluestone CD, Klein JO. *Impedance Screening for Middle Ear Disease in Children.* New York: Grune & Stratton; 1978.

Herrmann BS, Thornton AR, Joseph JM. Automated infant hearing screening using the abr: development and validation. In: Bess FH, Gravel JS, eds. *Foundations of Pediatric Audiology: A Book of Readings.* San Diego, CA: Plural Publishing; 2006.

Hayes D. State programs for universal newborn hearing screening. *Pediatr Clin North Am.* 1999;46:89–94.

Joint Committee on Infant Hearing 2000 Position Statement. *Principles and Guidelines for Early Hearing Detection and Intervention Programs.* Washington, DC: American Speech-Language-Hearing Association; 2000.

Kileny PR. ALGO-1 automated infant hearing screener: Preliminary results. In: Gerkin KP, Amochaev A, eds. *Hearing in Infants: Proceedings from the National Symposium. Seminars in Hearing.* New York: Thieme-Stratton; 1987.

Lous J. Screening for secretory otitis media: Evaluation of some impedance programs for long-lasting secretory otitis media in 7-year-old children. *Int J Pediatr Otorhinolaryngol.* 1987;13:85–97.

Matkin ND. Early recognition and referral of hearing-impaired children. *Pediatr Rev.* 1984;6:151–156.

Northern JL, Downs MP. *Hearing in Children.* 5th Ed. Baltimore: Lippincott Williams & Wilkins; 2002.

Nozza RJ, Bluestone CD, Kardatzke D, Bachman RN. Towards the validation of aural acoustic immittance measures for diagnosis of middle ear effusion in children. *Ear Hearing,* 1992;13:442–453.

Nozza RJ, Bluestone CD, Kardatzke D, Bachman RN. Identification of middle ear effusion by aural acoustic admittance and otoscopy. *Ear Hearing.* 1994;15:310–323.

Prieve B, Dalzell L, Berg A, et al. The New York State Universal Newborn Hearing Screening Demonstration Project: Outpatient outcome measures. In: Bess FH, Gravel JS. *Foundations of Pediatric Audiology: A Book of Readings.* San Diego, CA: Plural Publishing; 2006.

Roush J, Bryant K, Mundy M, Zeisel S, Roberts J. Developmental changes in static admittance and tympanometric width in infants and toddlers. *J Am Acad Audiol.* 1995;6,334–338.

Roush J. Screening school-age children. In Bess FH, Hall JW, eds. *Screening Children for Auditory Function.* Nashville: Bill Wilkerson Center Press; 1992.

Sackett DL, Haynes RB, Guyatt, GH, Tugwell P. *Clinical Epidemiology: A Basic Science for Clinical Medicine.* 2nd ed. Boston: Little Brown; 1991.

Stevens JC, Parker G. Screening and surveillance. In Newton VE, ed. *Paediatric Audiological Medicine.* London: Whurr Publishing; 2002.

Walton WK, Williams PS. Stability of routinely serviced portable audiometers. *Lang Speech Hear Services Schools.* 1972;3:36–43.

Weber BA. Screening of high-risk infants using auditory brainstem response audiometry. In Bess FH, ed. *Hearing Impairment in Children.* Parkton, MD: York Press; 1988.

Welsh R, Slater S. The state of infant hearing impairment identification programs. *ASHA.* 1993;35:49–52.

Wilson WR, Walton WK. Public school audiometry. In Martin FN, ed. *Pediatric Audiology.* Englewood Cliffs, NJ: Prentice-Hall; 1978.

ANSWERS TO PROBLEM IN VIGNETTE 6.2

Prevalence = 50%; Sensitivity = 80%; Specificity = 90%

Auditory Prosthetic Devices for People with Impaired Hearing

CHAPTER OBJECTIVES

- To understand the function of various auditory prosthetic devices, such as hearing aids, classroom amplification systems, and cochlear implants, devices which are designed to restore auditory perception to those individuals with impaired hearing;
- To recognize the differences between hearing aids, classroom amplification systems, assistive listening devices, and cochlear implants;
- To appreciate that the selection and fitting of the appropriate device is just the initial step in the process of aural rehabilitation; and
- To realize that, especially for school-aged children, maintenance of the auditory prosthetic device to ensure its function is critical to the successful use of the device.

KEY TERMS AND DEFINITIONS

- **Hearing aid**: A personal electroacoustic device, typically worn in or on the ear of persons with impaired hearing, which primarily serves to amplify sound arriving at the wearer's ear so as to compensate for the wearer's hearing loss.
- **Classroom amplification system**: An electroacoustic system typically making use of a detached microphone worn by the teacher with the microphone's output sent to personal amplification units worn by members of the class who have impaired hearing.
- **Assistive listening devices**: A wide assortment of electronic devices designed as either alternatives to or supplements of other auditory prosthetic devices. Depending on the severity of the hearing loss, common assistive listening devices include wireless systems designed

for use while watching television, systems for using the telephone, and the use of visual stimulation (e.g., flashing lights) for doorbells, alarm clocks, or other alerting devices.

- **Cochlear implant**: An electronic device that is surgically implanted under the skin behind the ear with electrodes (wires) extending through the middle ear and inserting into the fluid-filled cochlea. The normal transducer function of the inner ear is bypassed and the nerve fibers exiting the cochlea are stimulated directly by electrical current. These devices currently are reserved for use by individuals with severe or profound amounts of hearing loss who demonstrate little benefit from conventional hearing aids.

Hearing loss can result in a break in the communication chain that is in need of repair to restore normal communication. In the case of conductive pathology, the repair is often medical or surgical intervention to eliminate the pathology or disease causing the communication break. For individuals with sensorineural hearing loss from cochlear pathology, however, such medical repair is not possible. Instead, prosthetic devices are used to restore function to as close to normal as possible. Everyday examples of prosthetic devices used to restore function in other parts of the body include eyeglasses or contact lenses to correct visual problems and artificial limbs to compensate for the loss of a limb. In our case, however, we are specifically interested in prosthetic devices designed to compensate for hearing loss. Some of these devices, such as **hearing aids** or other amplification systems, primarily increase the intensity of sounds at the frequencies for which the person has hearing loss. These devices deliver more intense sounds to the outer ear and make use of the normal air-conduction transmission/transduction path from the middle ear to the inner ear. Alternatively, some devices are designed to bypass entirely the damaged portion of the normal auditory transmission/transduction path. A **cochlear implant**, for example, skips the outer ear, middle ear, and much of the inner ear by stimulating the auditory nerve fibers in the cochlea directly with electrical energy.

The reader should keep in mind that auditory prosthetic devices, such as hearing aids and cochlear implants, are typically used for persons with sensorineural hearing loss resulting from inner ear pathology. Although eyeglasses were mentioned as another common prosthetic device, this analogy often leads individuals to think that hearing is restored to "20/20" as soon as the hearing aid or cochlear implant has been fitted. This is often not the case in hearing, however, even following prolonged use of the devices, because the nature of the problem being treated in vision and in hearing is entirely different. Basically, in vision, the problems typically treated with eyeglasses (nearsightedness or farsightedness) are equivalent to *conductive* problems in hearing. Hearing aids work wonderfully with conductive impairments and can restore hearing to normal, but they are rarely used in such cases, as noted frequently in earlier chapters, because these hearing losses can be remedied medically or surgically. In fact, optometrists and ophthalmologists are turning increasingly to surgical corrections of nearsightedness and farsightedness, through procedures such as laser-assisted in-situ keratomileusis (LASIK), as alternatives to use of prosthetic devices for these vision problems. The overwhelming majority of persons using hearing aids or cochlear implants, however, do not have conductive hearing loss; rather, the problem lies in the auditory sensory receptors in the cochlea (the inner and outer hair cells). The visual analog to sensorineural hearing loss would be vision disorders that impact the sensory cells for vision—the rods and cones in the retina. When retinal damage is the source of the visual problem, as in vision disorders associated with macular degeneration, then prosthetic devices such as eyeglasses are generally incapable of restoring vision to "20/20."

Thus, although eyeglasses and hearing aids both represent prosthetic devices designed to assist individuals who have lost sensory function, the problems being treated with these devices are usually quite different and the expectations regarding benefits should be tempered accordingly. Sometimes, just making the hearing-impaired adult aware of the differences between eyeglasses and hearing aids, both in terms of the nature of the problem being treated by each and the expected benefits provided by each, can help the individual set realistic expectations and increase the odds for successful rehabilitation.

Given the foregoing, it is extremely rare for an individual with impaired hearing to receive maximum benefit as soon as the device is fitted. Instead, a period of adjustment, training, and rehabilitation is required. As a result, before we describe various prosthetic devices used by individuals with hearing impairment in detail, a broad overview of the aural rehabilitation process will put the use of these prosthetic devices in the proper context. The main point is that the intervention phase of rehabilitation, described briefly below, *begins*, rather than ends, with the fitting of the prosthetic device.

AN OVERVIEW OF THE AURAL REHABILITATION/ HABILITATION PROCESS

The aural rehabilitation process involves at least two phases. The first phase is the identification of the problem. Before an intervention strategy can be developed, one must know about the type and degree of hearing loss as well as the impact of the impairment on communicative, educational, social, or cognitive function. For the adult with hearing impairment, the measurement of the patient's audiogram, the administration of speech-recognition tests, and the use of self-report surveys or questionnaires can provide much of this information. Pure-tone and speech audiometry have already been discussed (Chapter 5). Self-report surveys are often used to assess in detail the social, psychologic, and communicative difficulties experienced by the hearing impaired. For the child with hearing impairment, additional assessment considerations might include the extent of parental support and the evaluation of skills in language, speech, auditory training, and speechreading (lipreading).

After the problem has been identified, the next phase of the rehabilitation process is intervention. For the hearing impaired, the nature of the intervention package is determined, in large part, by the identification phase. Consider, for example, just the degree and type of hearing loss, ignoring other factors such as age and social or emotional difficulties. First, regarding type of hearing loss, the most appropriate candidates for amplification are those with sensorineural hearing loss. Occasionally, individuals with chronic conductive hearing loss not amenable to medical or surgical intervention will be fitted with a hearing aid. For these individuals, a bone-anchored hearing aid that delivers sound to the inner ear via bone conduction is a viable option. Most often, though, the individual with sensorineural hearing loss as a result of cochlear pathology is the type of patient fitted with a rehabilitative device, such as a hearing aid.

Generally, as the degree of sensorineural hearing loss increases, speech-understanding difficulties increase. The need for intervention increases in proportion to the degree of speech-understanding difficulty. Thus, those with mild hearing loss (pure-tone average [PTA] of 20 to 30 dB HL) generally have less need for intervention than do those with profound hearing loss (PTA >85 dB HL). Conventional hearing aids provide the greatest benefit to those hearing-impaired persons whose average hearing loss is between 40 and 85 dB HL. For milder amounts of hearing loss, the difficulties experienced and the need for intervention often are not great enough for full-time use of a conventional hearing aid. Part-time use of a hearing aid, or another type of device known as an *assistive listening device*, is usually recommended for these patients. For the profoundly impaired, on the other hand, the difficulties in communicating and the need for intervention are great. Unfortunately, the conventional hearing aid is of limited benefit in such cases. For patients with profound impairments, alternative devices, such as cochlear implants, are explored. For patients with profound impairments fit with either high-powered hearing aids or cochlear implants, the fitting of the device is usually accompanied by extensive training in several areas, including speechreading (lipreading), auditory training, and/or manual communication (finger spelling and sign language).

Consider also the time of onset of the hearing loss. Of course, the intervention approach will be much different for a congenitally hearing-impaired child than for someone who acquired the hearing loss later in life (after communication has developed). With a congenital onset, the emphasis will focus on such critical issues as early intervention, parental guidance, and a comprehensive habilitation package designed to facilitate communication development.

In summary, the intervention phase of aural rehabilitation/habilitation typically begins with the selection and fitting of an appropriate rehabilitative device, such as a hearing aid or cochlear implant. This is followed by extensive training with the device in communicative situations.

Many of the procedures used in the identification phase of the rehabilitation process have been reviewed in earlier chapters. This chapter focuses on the devices available to hearing-impaired adults and children during the intervention phase, with emphasis on the conventional hearing aid and the cochlear implant. Chapter 8 focuses on the training methods and philosophies for rehabilitation/habilitation of children and adults once a device has been selected and fitted.

AMPLIFICATION FOR INDIVIDUAL WITH HEARING LOSS

Classification of Conventional Amplification

Today, the following six types of hearing aids are available: body aid, eyeglass aid, behind-the-ear (BTE) aid, in-the-ear (ITE) aid, in-the-canal (ITC) aid, and completely-in-the-canal (CIC) aid. Figure 7.1 shows the first five types of hearing aids, whereas the CIC hearing-aid type is illustrated in Vignette 7.1. When electroacoustic hearing aids were first developed several decades ago, the body aid was the only type available. In the ensuing years, the other types of instruments were developed. In 1960, eyeglass hearing aids were the most popular, accounting for 44% of all hearing aids sold, with the remaining 56% divided evenly between body and BTE instruments. As indicated in Figure 7.2, BTE hearing aids became the most common type of hearing aid sold in the two-decade period from 1962 through 1982. Since 1983, however, ITE aids have captured an increasingly larger portion of the hearing aid market. Since 1987, approximately 80% of the hearing aids sold in the United States have been ITE instruments; the bulk of the remaining 20% of instruments sold have been of the BTE type. Beginning in 2003, however, there has been a considerable upturn in the percentage of BTE hearing aids sold in the United States, increasing to about 40% in 2006, owing to new innovations in these devices and the resulting decrease in their visibility.

The sales percentages for ITEs shown in Figure 7.2 actually represent the combination of all types of ITE hearing aids, including the ITE, ITC, and CIC

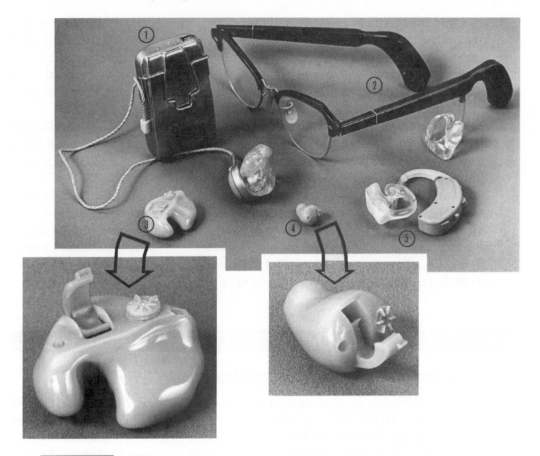

FIGURE 7.1   The different types of hearing aids. *1*, body aid; *2*, eyeglass; *3*, in-the-ear aid; *4*, in-the-canal aid; and *5*, behind-the-ear aid.

types. From 1995 through 2000, approximately 43% of the aids sold were custom ITE aids, most of which were full-concha devices, 22.5% were the ITC type, and 14.5% were the CIC type. Since 2000, the sales percentages for ITC and CIC types have remained about the same, but full-concha ITE hearing aids have decreased by 15% to 20% (to about 30% in 2005), about the same as the increase in BTE hearing aid sales over this same period. The increasing popularity of the less visible BTE, and the sustained popularity of the ITC and CIC hearing aids, is a result of both consumer pressures to improve the cosmetic appeal of the devices and rapid developments in the field of electronics. High-fidelity electronic components and the batteries to power them have been drastically reduced in size, making the smaller BTE and ITE devices possible.

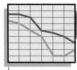

VIGNETTE 7.1 CLINICAL APPLICATION

The Completely-In-The-Canal (CIC) Hearing Aid

The drawing below depicts the size and position of a completely-in-the-canal (CIC) hearing aid in the ear canal of an adult hearing-aid wearer. The CIC hearing aid is the smallest commercially available hearing aid. As a result, it is the least conspicuous visually. Its small size, however, presents some special challenges to the audiologist, the wearer, and the manufacturer. First, for the manufacturer, the circuitry had to be miniaturized so as to have all components fit within this small space. In addition, given its small size and deep insertion, it is not possible to adjust controls on the hearing aid manually, as in other hearing aids. In most cases, manufacturers produce their CIC instruments with an electronic feature known as automatic volume control (AVC). The AVC circuit monitors the input level and gradually adjusts the gain to maintain a constant output level, much like the wearer would do with a manual volume control wheel. For the audiologist, two of the major challenges with such devices are the need for deep earmold impressions, because the device is designed to fit deeper within the ear canal than most other hearing aids, and the verification of a good fit with real-ear

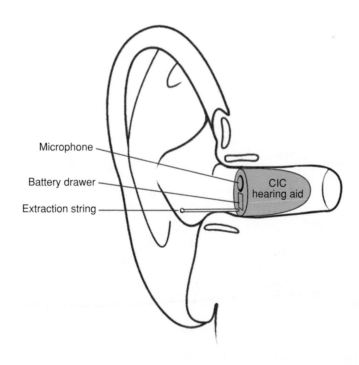

measurements. Finally, for the user, the primary adjustment is centered on the small size of the device. It is inserted and removed with a semirigid extraction string that is very small itself. Because the majority of hearing-aid users are elderly adults, many of whom have diminished manual dexterity, the insertion and removal of these tiny devices, as well as battery replacement and hearing-aid cleaning, can be challenging tasks for the user.

Since 1994, the average price of the CIC hearing aid has been approximately twice that of the BTE and full-shell ITE hearing aid and approximately 50% higher than the ITC hearing aid for the same electronic circuitry. In 2000, the percentage of hearing aids returned to the manufacturer for credit (that is, the wearer returned the hearing aids to the dispenser within the 30-day money-back trial period) was highest for the CIC type at 23%. The return rate for ITC hearing aids was 19.0% in 2000, whereas the return rate for full-shell ITE hearing aids was 15.3%. Return rates have remained fairly stable since 2000.

Incidentally, at one time, the industry apparently considered naming these hearing aids "totally-in-the-canal" (TIC) devices. However, it was probably considered inadvisable to tell people that they had just paid a fair amount of money for "a TIC in their ear"—the industry wisely opted for CIC instead.

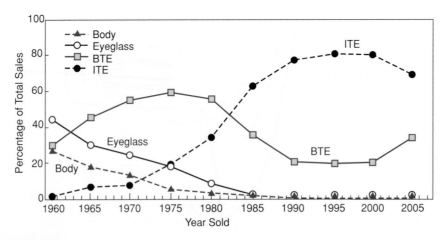

FIGURE 7.2 Sales trends for various hearing aid types since 1960. *BTE*, behind-the-ear; *ITE*, in-the-ear.

Operation of Amplification Systems

Components and Function

Although the outer physical characteristics of the types of hearing aids shown in Figure 7.1 differ, the internal features are very similar. The hearing aid, for example, is referred to as an *electroacoustic device*. It converts the acoustic signal, such as a speech sound, into an electrical signal. The device then manipulates the electrical signal in some way, converts the electrical signal back to an acoustic one, and then delivers it to the ear canal of the wearer. A microphone is used to convert the acoustic signal into an electrical signal. The electrical signal is usually amplified or made larger within the hearing aid. It may also be filtered to eliminate high or low frequencies from the signal. A tiny loudspeaker, usually referred to as a receiver, converts the amplified electrical signal back into a sound wave. Up to this point, the hearing aid could be thought of as a miniature public-address system with a microphone, amplifier, and loudspeaker. Unlike a public-address system, though, the hearing aid is designed to help a single person, the hearing-aid wearer, receive the amplified speech. The microphone is positioned somewhere on the hearing-aid wearer, and the amplified sound from the receiver is routed directly to the wearer's ear. For ITE and ITC hearing aids, the sound wave is routed from the receiver to the ear canal by a small piece of tubing within the plastic shell of the instrument. For the other types of hearing aids, an earmold is needed. The earmold (or shell for the ITE and ITC hearing aids) is made of a synthetic plastic or rubber-like material from an impression made of the outer ear and ear canal. The earmold is custom-made for the patient's ear and allows the output of the hearing aid to be coupled to the patient's ear canal. As a result, only the patient receives the louder sound and not a group of people, as with a public-address system (see Vignette 7.2).

Over 95% of the hearing aids sold in the United States in 2005 were digital devices. The amplifier referred to previously has basically been replaced by a small digital computer that can process the sound input received from the microphone prior to sending it to the loudspeaker or receiver. This change to digital circuitry has greatly expanded the options available to hearing aid manufacturers, audiologists and patients. The basic concept behind the hearing aid is the same and one of the primary purposes served by the digital processor is the amplification of sound, but the way in which this can be accomplished has been enhanced considerably.

Electroacoustic Characteristics of Hearing Aids

The primary purpose of the hearing aid is to make speech that is inaudible to the hearing-impaired person audible without causing discomfort. Modern-day

VIGNETTE 7.2   FURTHER DISCUSSION

Basic Components of an Electronic Hearing Aid

The top part of the schematic drawing shows the basic components of a contemporary electronic hearing aid. As illustrated here, the hearing aid is like a miniature head-worn public-address (PA) system with a microphone, amplifier, and loudspeaker (or receiver). The amplifier needs a portable power supply to do its job, and this is supplied by a battery. In addition, a volume control allows the user to adjust the loudness so that sound is comfortably loud in different environments. The microphone and receiver are known as transducers in that their primary job is to convert waveforms from one form of energy to another. The microphone, for example, converts sound waves into electrical voltage waveforms. The amplifier then makes this incoming electrical waveform larger, and the receiver converts it back to a sound wave.

   Although the components shown in the top portion of the drawing are fundamental to almost all electronic hearing aids, most hearing aids also come equipped with two additional controls. These are illustrated in the bottom portion of the drawing and are listed as the "tone control" and the "output limiting control." These two controls are generally adjusted by the audiologist and not by the hearing-aid wearer. The tone control functions like a bass or treble control on a stereo in that the audiologist can adjust it to change the amount of amplification in the low or high frequencies. The output-limiting control allows the audiologist to regulate the maximum possible sound level produced by the hearing aid to assure that loud sounds are not made uncomfortably or hazardously loud.

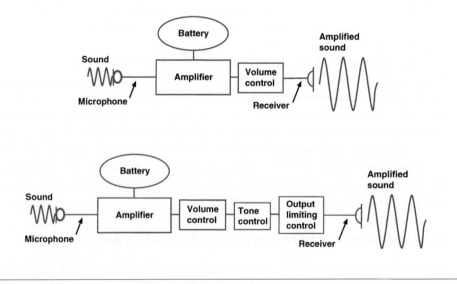

conventional hearing aids have several electroacoustic characteristics that are used to describe the hearing aid's performance. Probably the two most important of these characteristics are the amount of amplification provided, referred to as the gain of the instrument, and the maximum possible sound pressure level that can be produced, referred to as the maximum output. Currently, these characteristics can be measured in several ways. For instance, there is a standard issued by the American National Standards Institute, ANSI S3.22-2003, which describes a set of measurements that must be made on all hearing aids sold in the United States. It is not necessary in an introductory text such as this, however, to review the ANSI standard in detail. Rather, the concepts underlying gain and maximum output and their importance in fitting the hearing aid to the patient are critical.

Gain, for example, is simply the difference in decibels between the input level and the output level at a particular frequency. Consider the following example. A 500-Hz pure tone is generated from a loudspeaker so that the sound level at the hearing aid's microphone is 60 dB SPL. The output produced by the hearing aid under these conditions is 90 dB SPL. The acoustic gain provided by the hearing aid is 30 dB. The gain is simply the difference between the 60-dB SPL input and the 90-dB SPL output. The gain of the hearing aid can be measured at several frequencies. Most hearing aids provide some amplification or gain over the frequency range 200 Hz to at least 5,000 Hz. When the gain is measured across this whole frequency range by changing the frequency of the input signal and holding the input level constant, a frequency response for the hearing aid is obtained. The frequency response displays how the output or gain varies as a function of frequency. The concepts of gain and frequency response are illustrated in Figure 7.3. Because the gain is seldom constant at all frequencies, an average gain value is frequently calculated and reported. In the current ANSI standard, the gain is measured at three frequencies, 1,000, 1,600, and 2,500 Hz, and the values are averaged. These frequencies are used because of their importance to speech understanding and because the hearing aid usually has its greatest output in this frequency region.

A feature shared by many hearing aids is a volume control wheel that adjusts the gain of the hearing aid under manual control by the user. In many contemporary digital hearing aids, the adjustment of the volume is accomplished automatically by the digital processor. The frequency response of the hearing aid can be measured while the position of the volume control is varied, either manually or electronically. Usually, at least two sets of measurements are obtained: one with the volume control in the full-on position and one designed to approximate a typical or "as worn" volume setting. The volume control is designed to provide about a 30-dB variation in gain. It is typically

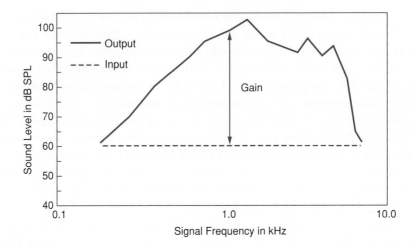

FIGURE 7.3 Calculation of hearing aid gain. The *output curve* represents the frequency response of the hearing aid for a constant 60-dB *input.*

assumed that a hearing-aid wearer will select a volume setting somewhere in the middle of this 30-dB range (i.e., approximately 15 dB below the full-on position). If the frequency response is measured with the volume control of the hearing aid in the full-on position, the gain is referred to as "full-on" gain. When the volume control is in the middle of the usable range, the gain approximates "use" gain, or "as worn" gain.

As mentioned, a second fundamental electroacoustic characteristic of the hearing aid is the maximum output. Maximum output is measured to determine the maximum possible acoustic output of the hearing aid. Consequently, a high-level input signal is used (90 dB SPL), and the volume control is set to the full-on position. Under these conditions, the hearing aid is likely to be at maximum output. The maximum output should be adjusted carefully by the audiologist to optimize the amount of gain available to the wearer while simultaneously minimizing the amount of time the hearing aid is in saturation during use.

The gain and maximum output of a hearing aid are interrelated, as illustrated in Figure 7.4. The function shown in this figure is known as an input-output function because it displays the output along the ordinate as a function of the input level along the abscissa. For this hypothetical input-output function, the volume control is assumed to be in the full-on position. Note that low input levels (50 to 60 dB SPL) reveal output values that exceed the input by 25 dB. The gain (output minus input) is 25 dB at low input levels. At high input levels (90 to 100 dB SPL), on the other hand, the output remains constant at 110 dB SPL. This is the maximum output of the hearing aid. The instrument is set so

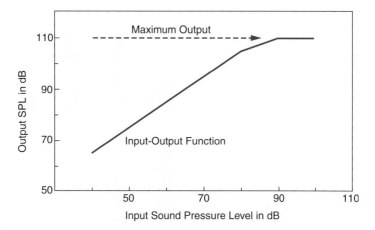

FIGURE 7.4 Input-output function for a hearing aid.

that it cannot produce an output higher than 110 dB SPL. Because the hearing aid is at maximum output, the gain at these higher input levels is lower. The gain for the 90- and 100-dB inputs is 20 and 10 dB, respectively. Because of this interaction between gain and maximum output, gain is usually measured for lower input levels (e.g., 50 dB SPL); levels that also approximate those of conversational speech, the input signal of greatest interest.

Over most of the range of input sound levels in Figure 7.4, every time the input was increased 10 dB, the output demonstrated a corresponding increase of 10 dB. This was true until the maximum output or saturation level of the hearing aid was reached. Such a circuit is generally referred to as a *linear circuit*. Many hearing aids dispensed today have intentionally nonlinear amplification circuits, often referred to as *compression circuits*, which are designed to obtain a better match between the wide range of sound levels in the environment and the narrower range of listening available in the hearing-impaired person.

Along with a wider range of possible settings and processing options associated with digital hearing aids, these devices often have multiple memories that can hold different combinations of settings. This allows the hearing-aid wearer to adjust the various settings of the hearing aid easily and quickly for specific listening situations, such as listening to the television alone at home or conversing with an acquaintance at a bustling restaurant.

Candidacy for Amplification

How does one know whether an individual is a good candidate for amplification? We have already indicated that the typical candidate for amplification is

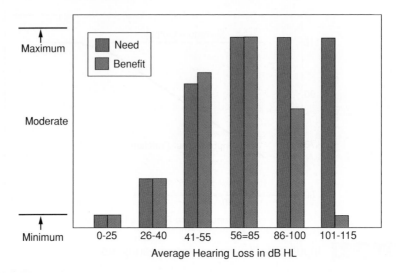

FIGURE 7.5 Illustration of the need for and potential benefit from amplification as a function of degree of hearing loss.

one who displays a sensorineural hearing loss. Many audiologists use the degree of hearing loss as a "rule of thumb" for determining hearing aid candidacy. Figure 7.5 shows a general guideline based on the average (500 to 2,000 Hz) pure-tone hearing loss in the better ear. As hearing loss increases, the need for assistance increases, reaching a maximum for moderate amounts of hearing loss. Potential benefit from amplification, however, is lowest at the two extremes of mild and profound impairment. Those individuals with the mildest hearing losses and those with the most profound hearing deficits are usually the candidates who will benefit the least from a hearing aid. There are many exceptions to this rule of thumb, which is based simply on pure-tone thresholds. Because of this, there is now a tendency to move away from these pure-tone guidelines and consider anyone with a communicative difficulty caused by hearing impairment as a candidate for amplification.

There are other considerations in determining hearing-aid candidacy. Some of these factors are the patient's motivation for seeking assistance, the patient's acceptance of the hearing loss, and the patient's cosmetic concerns. Even if a significant hearing loss is present, some older adults put off seeking assistance for several years. The reasons for this delay are not altogether clear, although the cost of the hearing aid and the failure of the primary-care physician to refer for a hearing aid are considered contributing factors. Factors that influence individuals to pursue amplification include communication problems at home, communication problems in noisy situations or in social settings, communication problems at work, and encouragement from a spouse or loved one.

Acceptance of a hearing loss is another consideration in determining hearing-aid candidacy. Some individuals simply deny that a hearing problem exists. This is particularly true for persons with very mild losses, those who fear loss of employment, and those who have suffered gradual onset of hearing loss.

Finally, one cannot overlook cosmetic concerns when considering a patient's candidacy for amplification. Amplification is still considered stigmatic. Although the acceptance of hearing aids is improving, many hearing-impaired individuals are concerned about the stigma associated with readily visible amplification devices. (This is discussed in more detail later in Vignette 8.1.)

Hearing-Aid Selection and Evaluation

Once it has been established that an individual can benefit from amplification, an appointment for hearing-aid selection and evaluation is usually scheduled. In the selection phase, some important clinical decisions must be made. For example, what type of hearing aid would be most appropriate for a given hearing-impaired person? Recall from Figure 7.1 that a number of different types of hearing aids are available. The audiologist and patient need to decide whether the patient will benefit most from a BTE instrument or one of the ITE systems (ITE, ITC, or CIC). As noted earlier, most hearing aids sold today are BTE, ITE, ITC, or CIC units. BTE hearing aids have several distinct advantages over earlier body aids, the most important of which are cosmetic appeal, improved sound localization, and better speech understanding in noise when two aids are worn. Importantly, very few young children wear ITE, ITC, or CIC systems because of the frequent need to recast the earpiece due to a growing ear canal. Currently, approximately 75% of hearing aids selected for children are BTE systems. #17

Another important clinical decision that must be made in the selection phase is whether to recommend one hearing aid (monaural amplification) or two hearing aids (binaural amplification). Decades ago, there had been considerable controversy over the true benefits of binaural amplification, but this is no longer the case. In 2006, 75% to 80% of hearing aids dispensed in the United States were binaural fittings. The primary reason why binaural amplification is not even more widespread is undoubtedly the added cost to the patient of buying two hearing aids rather than one. Nonetheless, there is mounting clinical evidence that failure to fit hearing aids on both ears of patients with bilateral hearing loss can result in temporary, and perhaps permanent, decreases in auditory function in the unaided ear. The deterioration over time of auditory perceptual function in the hearing-impaired ear left unaided has been referred to as an *auditory deprivation effect.*

In addition to avoiding these possible deprivation or adaptation effects, some of the reported advantages to binaural amplification include better sound localization, binaural summation (a sound is easier to hear with two ears than with one and the user can make use of lower volume settings as a result), and improvement in speech recognition in noise. Experienced hearing-aid users often favor binaural amplification and report that two aids offer more balanced hearing, better overall hearing, improved speech clarity in noise, improved sound localization skills, and more natural and less stressful listening. Accordingly, binaural amplification is being recommended with increasing regularity. Some clinical research indicates that the benefits of binaural fittings over monaural ones increase as the amount of hearing loss increases. Monaural fittings may be appropriate for many persons with mild hearing impairment.

Several other factors must be considered in the selection process but are beyond the scope of an introductory text. Briefly, the audiologist must consider the type of microphone (directional versus omnidirectional), earmold material (soft silastic versus hard acrylic), and type of earmold or shell (e.g., open versus vented versus unvented). For children, an additional consideration is the adaptability of the instrument to various classroom amplification systems.

Modern-day hearing aids provide a wide range of electroacoustic characteristics that can be tailored to the patient's individual needs. The process of selecting a hearing aid with the appropriate electroacoustic characteristics for a particular patient is referred to as hearing-aid selection. This process has undergone major changes in recent years. Today, most audiologists use a prescriptive approach to hearing-aid selection. Using information obtained from the patient, such as the pure-tone thresholds, the appropriate gain can be prescribed according to some underlying theoretical principles. From the mid-1970s through the mid-1980s, at least a dozen different prescriptive hearing-aid selection methods were developed. Although they differ in detail, these methods have the same general feature that more gain is prescribed at those frequencies for which the hearing loss is greatest. As an example, one of the simplest approaches makes use of the so-called *half-gain rule*. One simply measures the hearing threshold at several frequencies and multiplies the hearing loss by a factor of one half. Thus, for a patient with a flat 50-dB hearing loss from 250 to 8,000 Hz, the appropriate gain would be 25 dB (0.5×50 dB) at each frequency. A person having a sloping hearing loss with a 40-dB HL hearing threshold at 1,000 Hz and an 80-dB HL threshold at 4,000 Hz would require gains of 20 and 40 dB, respectively, using this simple one-half gain rule. Regardless of the prescriptive method used, once the prescription is made, the audiologist searches among existing hearing aids capable of producing the desired gain and maximum output at each frequency and then programs the digital processor accordingly.

Maximum output can also be prescribed for the patient. Usually, additional information is required from the patient. One common approach is to measure the loudness discomfort level (LDL) of the patient for tones or narrow bands of noise. The LDL is a measure of the maximum sound level that the patient can tolerate at each frequency. When it is not possible to measure loudness discomfort levels at several frequencies in each ear, as with most young children, LDLs can be estimated from pure-tone thresholds. It would not be desirable for the hearing aid's acoustic output to exceed the maximum tolerable level of the patient because this might cause the patient to reject the hearing aid. The maximum output of the hearing aid is frequently adjusted to a value slightly lower than the LDL. In this way, the audiologist can be assured that the acoustic output of the hearing aid will not exceed the maximum tolerance level of the patient. As noted, many modern hearing aids have intentionally nonlinear input-output functions so that the gain available steadily decreases as the input level increases. Although these hearing aids require different prescription procedures than linear hearing aids, the basic process is very similar regardless of the type of hearing-aid circuit.

Once the appropriate prescription has been made and the hearing aid has been selected, the next process, the hearing aid fitting, is conducted. In this #18 process, the hearing aid is inserted into the patient's ear and its acoustic performance on the wearer is verified. This is most commonly accomplished using real-ear measurements of the sound pressure level generated in the ear canal, in close proximity to the eardrum, with and without the hearing aid in place. This is made possible by using a tiny microphone connected to a long, thin tube made of flexible plastic. The tube can be safely inserted into the ear canal, yet it is strong enough to resist being squeezed shut when the hearing aid is inserted into the ear canal over the thin tube. When sound pressure level measurements are made at several frequencies in the patient's ear canal with and without the hearing aid, the difference between these two measurements provides a measure of the real-ear insertion gain of the hearing aid (Vignette 7.3). The measured insertion gain is compared with the target gain generated by the particular prescriptive method chosen by the audiologist (e.g., half-gain rule), and the hearing aid's settings are adjusted until a reasonable match is observed. Similar adjustments should also be made in the maximum output of the hearing aid to assure that real-ear sound pressure levels measured in the aided conditions for high-level input signals (90 dB SPL) do not exceed the LDL. Today, in many cases, rather than expressing targets in relative gain measured in the ear canal of the hearing-aid wearer, prescriptive procedures will specify the sound pressure levels that should be met for speech-like sounds when measured in the ear canal.

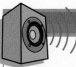

VIGNETTE 7.3   CONCEPTUAL DEMO

MEASUREMENT OF REAL-EAR INSERTION GAIN

As noted in the text, the measurement of real-ear insertion gain is a common first step in the verification of the fit of the hearing aid. The drawing below illustrates the basic arrangement of equipment needed for this measurement. Basically, a small loud-speaker is located at ear level about 1 m from the patient (either straight ahead or at a slight angle). A long, very narrow, flexible tube, referred to as the probe tube, is inserted into the ear canal. The closed end of the probe tube terminates at a

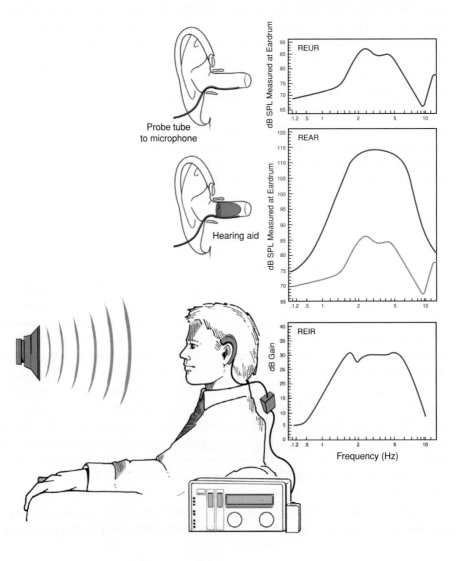

microphone, and the microphone is connected to the real-ear-measurement device. This device sends stimuli to the loudspeaker and records the measurements made with the microphone at the end of the probe tube. (Often, another microphone is attached to the side of the patient's head to monitor and regulate the output level of the loud-speaker at the patient's ear.)

The top panel above illustrates the position of the probe tube in the ear canal for the initial unaided measurements. When the sound is presented from the loudspeaker as a series of 60-dB SPL pure tones increasing in frequency from 100 to 10,000 Hz and measured in the open ear canal with the probe tube, a frequency response like that shown in the top panel is obtained. This is referred to as the real-ear unaided response (REUR). It shows the 15- to 20-dB resonant boost provided by the ear canal and pinna (Chapter 3). The middle panel above shows the next measurement made with the hearing aid inserted and adjusted to the appropriate settings. Sound is again presented from the loudspeaker as a series of 60-dB SPL pure tones increasing in frequency from 100 to 10,000 Hz. The sound levels recorded with the probe-tube microphone in the aided condition are referred to as the real-ear aided response (REAR).

The lower panel shows the difference between the REAR and REUR curves and is referred to as the real-ear insertion response or REIR. Essentially, this curve shows how much real-ear insertion gain (REIG) was provided, in dB, at each frequency from 100 to 10,000 Hz as a result of hearing-aid insertion. If the REIR was flat at 0 dB, for example, this would imply that there was no gain provided by the hearing aid. The audiologist compares the REIR to target values generated by various prescription procedures and fine tunes the hearing aid until the REIR demonstrates a close match to the target values. The REIR is a reliable measure, can be obtained in a matter of minutes, provides a very detailed picture of the hearing aid's response on that particular patient, and requires no active participation on the part of the hearing-aid wearer. It has become a very common and powerful tool for the verification of a hearing aid's performance on an individual wearer.

After fine-tuning the gain and maximum output of the hearing aid to match the targeted values, the hearing aid is evaluated. Again, there are several hearing-aid evaluation procedures from which the audiologist can choose. These alternatives, however, have a common goal: evaluation of the benefit provided by the hearing aid when it is worn by the hearing-impaired patient. Because the primary benefit to be derived from use of the hearing aid is improved understanding of speech, the hearing-aid evaluation usually involves the measurement of the patient's speech-recognition performance with and without the hearing aid. The patient is typically presented with a sample of continuous speech or speech-shaped noise at a level approximating conversational levels (65 or 70 dB SPL). While listening to this stimulus, the patient adjusts the volume control on the hearing aid to a comfortable setting. Next, speech-recognition testing is conducted, with the materials being presented at the same overall level (65 to 70 dB SPL). Speech-recognition testing is often performed both in quiet and in a background of noise to permit evaluation of the benefit provided by the hearing aid for a range of conditions representative of those in which the hearing aid is to be worn. The speech-recognition measures are also often obtained from the patient in quiet and in noise under identical stimulus conditions without the hearing aid. The difference in performance between the aided and unaided measures provides a general indication of the benefit provided by the hearing aid under various listening conditions. These direct measures of the effects of the hearing aid on speech-recognition performance have sometimes been referred to as "objective" measures of benefit.

In addition to these objective measures of hearing-aid benefit, the hearing-aid evaluation should also include some "subjective" measures of performance and benefit. Most commonly, self-assessment surveys or inventories of hearing handicap and hearing aid performance have been used with adults.

Hearing-Aid Orientation

Hearing aids are typically sold in the United States on a 30-day trial basis; dissatisfied patients are given a refund at the end of that trial period. During the trial period, the patient is encouraged to visit the audiologist two or three times for a series of hearing-aid orientations. During the hearing-aid orientations, the patient is instructed in the use and care of the hearing aid, counseled about its limitations, given strategies to maximize its benefit, and given an opportunity to voice any complaints about its function. Frequently, modification of the earmold or the earpiece (shell) of the aid is needed to make the hearing aid fit more comfortably in the patient's ear. The hearing aid may require some electronic adjustments as well. After the 30-day trial period, the hearing-aid user is encouraged to return for further evaluation in a year, or sooner if he or she experiences difficulty.

ALTERNATIVE PROSTHETIC DEVICES

Assistive Listening Devices

As mentioned previously, full-time use of a hearing aid is not necessary or beneficial for many hearing-impaired individuals. A number of adults with mild hearing loss require only part-time use of a hearing aid or alternative device.

For many of these individuals, a practical alternative is a class of devices known as **assistive listening devices**. These devices are typically electroacoustic devices designed with a much more limited purpose in mind than that of the conventional hearing aid. Two of the most common purposes for which these devices were developed include use of the telephone and listening to the television. Several telephone handsets have been developed, for instance, that can amplify the telephone signal by 15 to 30 dB. These devices are effective for adults with mild hearing loss who have difficulty communicating over the telephone.

Many of the assistive listening devices physically separate the microphone from the rest of the device so that the microphone can be placed closer to the source of the desired sound. Recall that the microphone converts an acoustic signal into an electrical one so that it can be amplified by the device. If the microphone on the assistive listening device is separated by a great distance from the rest of the device, then the electrical signal from the microphone must somehow be sent to the amplifier. This is accomplished in various ways. Some devices simply run a wire, several feet in length, directly from the microphone to the amplifier. Other devices convert the electrical signal from the microphone into radio waves (FM) or invisible light waves (infrared) and send the signal to a receiver adjacent to the amplifier and worn by the individual. The receiver converts the FM or infrared signal back to an electrical signal and sends it to the amplifier to be amplified.

The FM and infrared systems are frequently referred to as *wireless systems* because they eliminate the long wire running directly from the microphone to the amplifier. The wireless feature of these assistive listening devices makes them more versatile and easier to use, but it also makes them more expensive. These assistive listening devices overcome the primary disadvantage of the conventional hearing aid; they improve the speech-to-noise ratio. By separating the microphone from the rest of the device and positioning it closer to the sound source (e.g., the talker's mouth or the loudspeaker of the television set), the primary signal of interest is amplified more than the surrounding background noise. On a conventional hearing aid, the ear-level microphone amplifies both the speech and the surrounding noise equally well; therefore, the speech-to-noise ratio is not improved, and all sound at the position of the microphone is simply made louder by the conventional hearing aid (see Vignette 7.4).

Separating the microphone from the rest of the device, however, has its drawbacks. It is only a reasonable alternative when the sound source is fairly stable over time. If the microphone is positioned near the loudspeaker of the television, for example, the voice of a talker seated next to the impaired person will not be amplified. The impaired individual is forced to listen to the sound source closest to the microphone (the television, in this example). For assistive listening devices, this is not a serious drawback because they have a limited purpose.

VIGNETTE 7.4 FURTHER DISCUSSION

EFFECTS OF A HEARING AID ON SPEECH UNDERSTANDING IN QUIET AND IN NOISE

The *left-hand panel* in the figure a high-frequency sensorineural hearing loss, not unlike that found in many elderly individuals, has been superimposed on the speech audiogram. Notice that many of the high-frequency, low-intensity consonants are no longer heard by the individual with this hearing loss, although many low- and mid-frequency speech sounds (such as vowels and nasal sounds) remain audible. As noted previously, a frequent complaint of individuals with this very common type of hearing loss is that they can hear speech but they cannot understand it.

In the *right-hand panel*, the speech sounds have been amplified by a well-fit hearing aid. In this case, a well-fit hearing aid would amplify the high frequencies to make the high-frequency consonants audible to the patient while not amplifying the low frequencies, where hearing is essentially normal. With the audibility of all of the speech sounds in conversational speech restored by the hearing aid as shown in this panel, the hearing-aid wearer will regain the ability to understand speech as well as a normal-hearing listener. Depending, in part, on how long they have become accustomed to hearing speech through their hearing loss, the time required to perform normally will vary from patient to patient.

In noise, however, the microphone of the hearing aid amplifies the noise as much as the speech; thus, the speech-to-noise ratio is not improved by the conventional hearing aid. If the conversational speech of the person in front of the listener is 6 dB greater at the input to the hearing aid (microphone) than the background of babble produced by the other attendees at a cocktail party, then this 6-dB speech-to-noise ratio will remain at the output from the hearing aid. The speech will be made audible by the hearing aid but so will the noise. Consequently, conventional hearing aids are generally not considered to work as well in noise as in quiet.

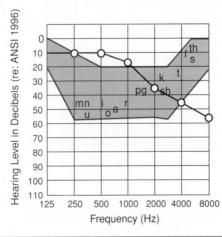

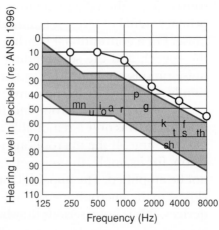

Selection and evaluation of assistive listening devices is not as formalized as it is for hearing aids. Many clinics today have a room designated as the "assistive listening device area." This room or area is set up to simulate the conditions under which the devices are to be used. Typically, the room takes on the atmosphere of a living room or family room, with television, stereo, and telephones available. After the patient's needs have been assessed through a written or oral questionnaire, several assistive devices are tried by the patient under controlled conditions in the simulated environment. If the patient finds the device beneficial, it is dispensed by the audiologist or the patient is referred to an appropriate source for its purchase.

Assistive devices of various types also benefit the severely or profoundly impaired. In addition to those devices mentioned above, some nonauditory devices have been developed. Devices have been produced that flash lights in response to various acoustic signals occurring in the home, such as the ringing of the doorbell or the telephone. Other special telephone devices enable text to be sent over phone lines (in printed form) so that a profoundly impaired person can carry on a telephone conversation by sending and receiving text messages. Special keyboard-like devices are needed at both ends of the phone line to enable such communication.

Classroom Amplification

A discussion of hearing aids would not be complete without a review of the special amplification systems designed for education. **Classroom amplification** is a term used to describe a hearing-aid device that provides amplified sound to a group of children while in the classroom. Classroom amplification gained added importance with the advent of a federal mandate regarding the education of all handicapped children. The law required that schools provide hearing-impaired children with adequate services and funding. This included habilitative/rehabilitative services, such as selection and evaluation of personal hearing aids and group systems, auditory training, speech training, speechreading, and any other services deemed necessary for the child's educational development.

Why should a child need a special educational amplification system? A primary concern is the acoustic environment that children are exposed to in the classroom. Children are continually bombarded with excessively high noise levels that interfere with their ability to understand the teacher. These noise levels originate from sources outside the school building (aircraft or car traffic), within the school building (adjacent classrooms and hallways, activity areas, heating/cooling systems), and within the classroom itself (students talking, feet shuffling, noise from moving furniture). These various noise sources contribute to noise levels ranging from 40 to 67 dBA. Such high noise levels result in an unfavorable signal-to-noise (S:N) or speech-to-noise ratio reaching the child's ear. Recall that a S:N ratio represents the difference, in decibels, between speech (from the teacher) and the overall ambient noise (within the classroom). For example, a S:N ratio of +10 dB means that the teacher's speech is 10 dB more intense than the noise in the classroom. Ideally, a S:N ratio of +20 dB is necessary if a child with hearing loss is to understand speech maximally. Noise surveys in classrooms have shown that S:N ratios typically range from −6 dB to +6 dB, a listening environment that precludes maximal understanding even for normal-hearing children.

Classroom noise is not the only variable that contributes to a difficult listening environment. *Reverberation time*, a term used to denote the amount of time it takes for sound to decrease by 60 dB after the termination of a signal, also contributes to an adverse acoustic environment. When a teacher talks to the child, some of the speech signal reaches the child's amplification system within just a few milliseconds. The remainder of the signal, however, strikes surrounding areas and reaches the child's ear after the initial sound in the form of reflections. The strength and duration of these reflections are affected by the absorption quality of the surrounding surfaces and the size (volume) of the classroom. If an area has hard walls, ceilings, and floors, the room will have a long reverberation time. In contrast, an acoustically treated room with carpeting, drapes, and an acoustic tile ceiling will have a shorter reverberation time. Generally, as reverberation time increases, the proportion of reflected speech sound reaching the listener increases and speech recognition decreases. In addition, the smaller the room size, the greater the reverberation. Many classrooms for the hearing-impaired have reverberation times ranging from a very mild value of 0.2 s to more severe reverberation, with times greater than 1 s.

These factors, noise and reverberation, are known to adversely affect speech recognition. As the noise levels and reverberation times increase, the S:N ratio becomes less favorable and there is a significant breakdown in speech understanding. Further, as the distance between the talker and listener increases, the S:N ratio worsens. Figure 7.6 illustrates this phenomenon.

Children with hearing loss not only experience difficulty understanding speech under difficult listening situations, but they also expend a great deal of effort in attending to the spoken message. Studies have demonstrated that not only does the presence of noise increase learning effort it even reduces the energy available for performing other cognitive functions. Even young school-aged children with very mild forms of hearing loss

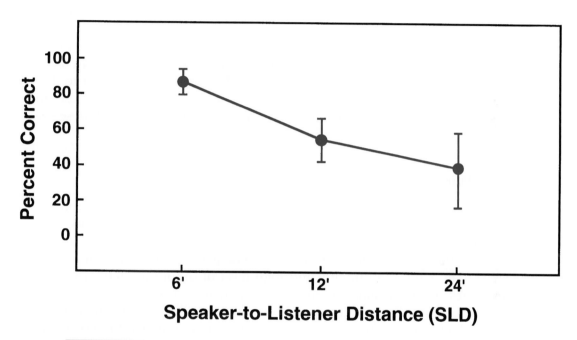

FIGURE 7.6 Typical speech-recognition scores for normal-hearing children at different speaker-to-listener distances. At 6 feet, the signal-to-noise ratio is +6 dB and the reverberation time is 0.46 s.

have reported less energy or were tired more frequently than children with normal hearing. These findings may well be a result of the difficulties these children experience listening under adverse listening conditions. One can speculate that toward the end of a school day, children with hearing loss will be physically and mentally "spent" as a result of focusing so intently on the teacher's speech and on the conversations of other children. This expenditure of effort will no doubt compromise a child's ability to learn in the classroom.

Several types of special educational amplification systems have been designed to overcome the adverse effects of the classroom environment by offering a better S:N ratio (Vignette 7.5). These system types include hard-wire systems, FM wireless systems, infrared systems, and a system that combines the FM wireless system with a personal hearing aid. More recently, sound-field amplification systems have been developed as yet another option for use in the classroom and one that may benefit *all* students in the classroom, not just those with hearing impairment. The concept behind these systems is similar to that described for the assistive listening devices. The microphone is moved closer to the desired sound source, the teacher. A brief description of each of these systems follows.

Hard-Wire System

In this system, a microphone worn by the teacher is wired to an amplifier. Each student then wears headphones or insert-type receivers that are connected to the amplifier by wires so that the teacher and the students are, in effect, "tethered" together (Fig. 7.7, *top*). The primary advantage of a hard-wire system is the high fidelity and high level of output available through earphones. These systems are inexpensive and are simple and easy to operate. The obvious disadvantage is the restricted mobility of both the teacher and students. Hard-wire systems are not very commonplace in classrooms today.

FM Wireless Systems

Most classrooms for the hearing-impaired use either FM devices or a combination of an FM system and a personal hearing aid. A microphone transmitter is worn around the teacher's neck, and a signal is broadcast to an FM receiver worn by the child (Fig. 7.7, *bottom*). Most FM receivers have an environmental microphone so that the child can monitor his or her own voice, the voices of his or her peers, and other environmental sounds. When the environmental microphone is used, however, the S:N ratio is compromised because of the distance between the talker and the microphone. The advantage to this system is the mobility allowed. In other words, the teacher and the students are free to move around the room and the students will continue to receive amplification.

VIGNETTE 7.5   FURTHER DISCUSSION

IMPROVING THE SPEECH-TO-NOISE RATIO WITH AN ASSISTIVE LISTENING DEVICE OR CLASSROOM SYSTEM

In this vignette, we will make use of the same "speech audiogram" concept used in Vignette 7.4. The top left-hand panel below shows the speech audiogram for conversational speech with a background noise (several other people talking) as it has been amplified by a hearing aid. This is the same as the right-hand panel of Vignette 7.4 with the addition of background noise. The level of the noise is indicated by the *blue dashed line*. The speech and noise levels shown here represent those measured through the hearing aid with the listener in the middle of a living room or classroom full of people at about 1 m from the desired talker.

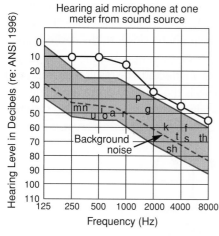

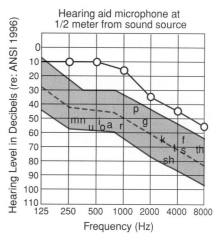

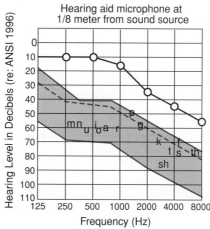

In the *top right panel*, the microphone has been detached from the hearing aid and is now positioned about half a meter from the primary talker. (The hearing aid's microphone really can't be detached. We're just pretending that it is to illustrate the concept behind assistive listening devices.) As the distance to the sound source is halved (from 1 m to a half meter), the sound level increases by 6 dB. Notice that the speech is now 6 dB higher than it was in the *left-hand panel*, whereas the diffuse background noise (*dashed line*) coming from a variety of sources, including reflections from walls and the ceiling, remains unchanged. Thus, the speech-to-noise ratio has improved 6 dB.

In the *bottom panel*, we have positioned the microphone still closer to the sound source, approximately one-eighth of a meter (4 to 5 inches) from the primary talker's mouth. As a result, the speech level from the talker has increased another 12 dB (two more halvings of the distance), and the speech-to-noise ratio has been improved a total of 18 dB compared with that in the *left-hand panel*.

As noted in Vignette 7.4, the conventional hearing aid does not improve the signal-to-noise ratio but simply amplifies the acoustic signals, speech and noise alike, that arrive at the microphone (*top left panel*). By moving the microphone closer to the desired sound source (*top right* and *bottom panels*), whether a talker or a loudspeaker, the speech signal level is increased while the background noise remains unaffected. The result is an improved speech-to-noise ratio and better communication. This is the primary operational principle behind many assistive listening devices, as well as similar classroom-amplification systems.

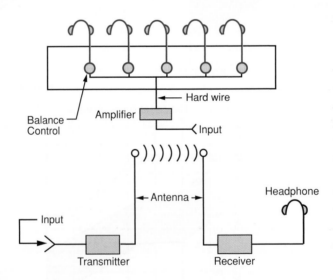

FIGURE 7.7 Two classroom amplification systems. *Top*, Hard-wire. *Bottom*, FM. The personal hearing aid could replace the headphones shown at bottom to produce a dovetailed system.

Infrared Systems

Infrared group amplification is seldom used in classroom settings but is used widely as an assistive device in theaters, churches, and other public facilities. As mentioned earlier, the system uses an infrared emitter that transmits the speech signal from the input microphone to individually worn infrared-receiver/audio-amplifier units. It is very similar in design to the FM system shown in Figure 7.7 (*bottom*), except that infrared light waves are used to send the signal from the transmitter to the receiver rather than FM radio waves. Infrared systems, however, are somewhat limited in power output.

Coupling the FM Wireless System to the Child's Ear

With personal FM systems, the teacher wears a microphone/transmitter that broadcasts carrier waves to a receiver worn by the child. A number of options are available for coupling the FM system to the child's ear. A summary of the coupling options that can be used with FM systems is shown in Vignette 7.6.

#15 & #16

Sound-Field Amplification

A more recent development in this area has been to broadcast the signal from the teacher's transmitter via FM transmission to an amplifier connected to a series of loudspeakers placed strategically around the classroom (Figure 7.8). Often, the loudspeakers are suspended from the ceiling, with at least two loudspeakers in the front and two at the rear of the classroom. The basic idea is that, through the presentation of the teacher's voice from loudspeakers dispersed throughout the classroom, no student is too far from the primary signal (the teacher's voice), and a favorable S:N is maintained throughout the classroom. Thus, the amplified signal is delivered uniformly to *all* students, rather than just those with hearing impairment. This can prove to be of benefit to not just other students with special needs but to normal-hearing children as well. As noted previously, the acoustics in many classrooms are poor and even normal-hearing children may find listening a challenge at times.

Similar to other amplification devices, the sound-field system has limitations: the amount of amplification is limited (8 to 10 dB) and the system amplifies only the teacher's voice, not the voices of other children. Of course, the hearing-impaired child can receive additional benefit from the use of a personal hearing aid in a classroom equipped with sound-field amplification. The low cost of the system and its potential to benefit many students in the classroom, however, make it an attractive alternative for many schools.

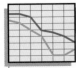

VIGNETTE 7.6   CLINICAL APPLICATIONS

METHODS OF COUPLING THE FM SYSTEM TO THE CHILD'S EAR

Several options exist for coupling the FM system to the ear. One option is to simply combine the FM device to the personal hearing aid. This approach, commonly referred to as *dovetailing*, is done to take advantage of the benefits of both systems: the improved speech-to-noise ratio offered by the FM system and the custom fitting of the personal

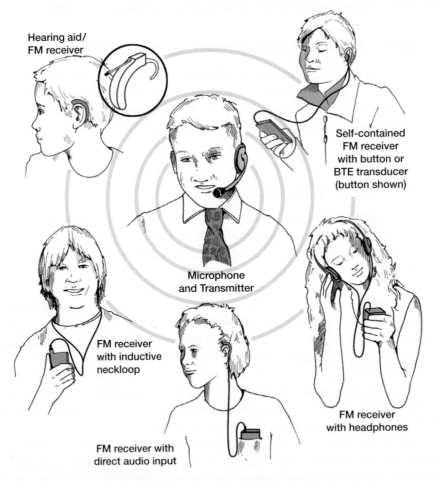

Hearing aid/
FM receiver

Self-contained
FM receiver
with button or
BTE transducer
(button shown)

Microphone
and Transmitter

FM receiver
with inductive
neckloop

FM receiver
with headphones

FM receiver with
direct audio input

(Figure adapted from Lewis DE. Classroom amplification. In Bess FH, ed: *Children with Hearing Impairment: Contemporary Trends*. Nashville: Bill Wilkerson Center Press; 1998, with permission.)

hearing aid. One approach for combining the FM system with the personal hearing aid is the incorporation of an FM receiver into an audio boot. When the boot is slipped on to an appropriate hearing aid, FM reception is possible. Some boots use an electrical connection from the student-worn receiver to the hearing aid; some manufacturers have developed wireless boots. Another approach to coupling a personal hearing aid to the FM system is via inductive coupling. With this device, the FM signal, which is sometimes mixed with an environmental signal within the student receiver, is converted to an electromagnetic field via a wire loop encircling the child's neck. The personal hearing aid is worn in the telecoil position, thereby inductively coupling a hearing aid to the FM receiver/mini-loop combination. A third approach is the use of a BTE FM receiver, a development brought about through advances in microminiature FM technology. The BTE houses, at ear level, both the FM receiver and the hearing aid circuitry, thus eliminating the need for cords, neckloops, and body-worn receivers. The BTE FM system device looks like a conventional BTE hearing aid. Other techniques for coupling the FM receiver to the child's ear include an FM system receiver with Sony Walkman type earbuds/headphones or simply a self-contained FM receiver with a button or BTE transducer.

A number of other populations known to experience difficulty under classroom-type noise conditions may also receive benefit from sound-field amplification. These populations include young children under the age of 15 years, children with articulation disorders, children with language disorders, children who are learning disabled, non-native English speakers, children with

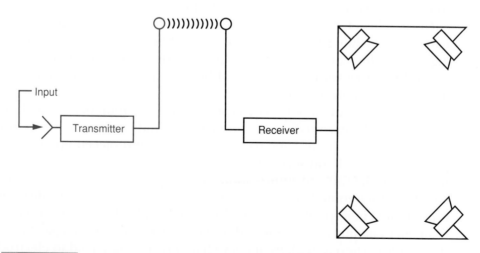

FIGURE 7.8   Diagram of a sound-field amplification system.

central auditory processing deficits, and children with a history of middle ear disease with effusion.

Cochlear Implants

In the 1980s, the cochlear implant emerged as a viable alternative to conventional amplification for individuals with profound hearing impairment. Several types of cochlear implants are available commercially today. They all share a common conceptual framework, but differ in its implementation. The cochlear implant is a device that is surgically implanted, with its stimulating electrode array (wire) inserted directly into the cochlea. The implant contains from 1 to 22 channels. Although individuals with the earlier single-channel cochlear implants may still be encountered by the clinician, all contemporary devices make use of multiple electrode arrays. The electrode is used to stimulate the auditory nerve directly with electric current, bypassing the damaged cochlear structures. As in the conventional hearing aid, a microphone is used to convert the acoustic signal into an electrical one. The electrical signal is then amplified and processed in various ways in a separate, body-worn component known as the *processor* or *stimulator*. The stimulator is about the size of a body-worn hearing aid or a package of cigarettes. Most recently, however, the stimulator and microphone have been combined into one ear-level unit, very similar to a BTE hearing aid. The output of the processor or stimulator is then sent to an external receiver worn behind the ear. This external receiver activates a similar internal receiver implanted surgically just under the skin and behind the ear. The implanted internal receiver converts the received signal into an electrical one and directs it to the electrode array penetrating the cochlea. This electrical signal, when routed to the electrode array, stimulates the remaining healthy auditory nerve fibers of the damaged inner ear. Figure 7.9 illustrates a typical arrangement for a cochlear implant and compares this device with a conventional hearing aid. As can be seen, these two devices share many features.

As noted, contemporary cochlear implants are multiple-channel devices. The "channels" essentially refer to adjacent bands in the frequency domain analogous to a series of band-pass filters. The sound picked up by the microphone is analyzed and sorted into several frequency-specific packets of information, or channels of information, by the processor. The output of each channel is then routed to a corresponding electrode in the electrode array that is positioned in a specific location along the length of the cochlea. Thus, low-frequency channels are connected to electrodes in the more apical region of the cochlea, whereas high-frequency channels are connected to electrodes in more basal locations. This system is an attempt to restore tonotopic mapping (Chapter 3) to the damaged cochlea.

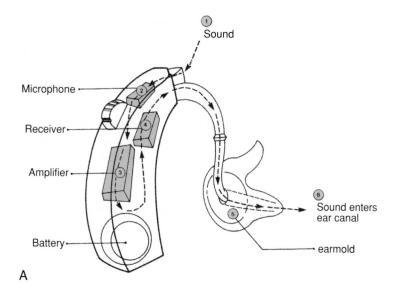

Sound ①

Microphone ②

Receiver ④

Amplifier ③

Battery

Sound enters ⑥
ear canal

earmold ⑤

A

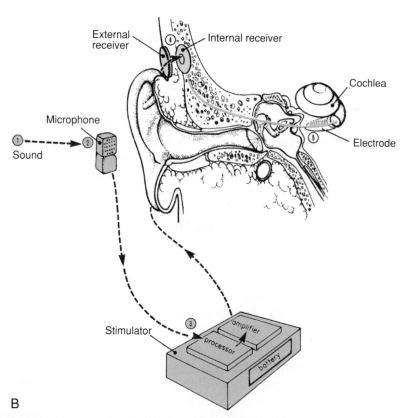

External receiver ④

Internal receiver

Cochlea

Microphone ②

Sound ①

Electrode ⑤

Stimulator ③

amplifier

processor

battery

B

FIGURE 7.9 Illustration of the similarities between conventional behind-the-ear hearing aid (*A*) and cochlear implant device (*B*). The components of each system are numbered identically to highlight the similarities.

For older children and adults, the *ideal* candidates for cochlear implants are those persons who acquired profound bilateral sensorineural hearing loss after acquiring language. Cochlear implants, however, appear to hold even greater promise for profoundly impaired prelingual children under 2 or 3 years of age, although research regarding the comparative benefits of rehabilitative devices in this population is still in progress. Although the results of clinical trials with these devices have varied markedly between patients, the best performance has been achieved with the multichannel devices implanted at the earliest ages. There are examples of "star" patients who perform remarkably well with the device without any visual cues and do so almost immediately. At a minimum, just about every recipient benefits from the device as an aid to speechreading and by increased awareness of sound. Its primary usefulness as an aid to speechreading seems to lie in making gross cues of timing and voicing available to the patient. Great strides continue to be made in the devices and in the training programs after implantation such that implants are the rehabilitative device of choice for the profoundly impaired, especially if implanted at an early age before the acquisition of language. Benefits of cochlear implantation have also been demonstrated in individuals with severe hearing loss as well, although the superiority of the implant to the hearing aid for severe hearing loss is less established.

The cochlear implant is intended to be a permanent, long-term solution to an extreme break (profound sensorineural hearing loss) in the communication chain. Compared to the cost of hearing aids, cochlear implants are 40 to 50 times more expensive (at least in terms of initial device purchase). Due to their expense, permanence, and irreversible destruction of any residual sensory structures in the cochlea, it would be beneficial to know the likelihood that a cochlear implant would be successful in a particular person *prior* to implantation. Such predictions are perhaps of greatest value for young children who have yet to acquire a language system. This has been an active area of research in recent years and progress continues to be made in identifying critical factors impacting the successful use of cochlear implants by children. For example, research published in 2003 identified several factors that increased the likelihood for a successful outcome with cochlear implants. Regarding the person receiving the implant, the likelihood of success with cochlear implants was enhanced for those young children who were female, had higher intelligence quotients (IQs), and were from smaller families with higher socioeconomic status. Of these factors, perhaps the only one that is somewhat surprising is the implant recipient's sex. Smaller families with more money have both the time and financial resources to provide the necessary intensive and extensive follow-up training that is needed. In addition, a higher IQ most likely reflects a better capability of the recipient's brain to make use of this new sensory code. In addition to these characteristics of the child or his or her family, factors associated with the devices themselves and the educational setting of the child were also identified that increased the odds for a successful outcome. Regarding the device, the greater the number of active electrodes, the better the child's performance with the implant. Regarding the educational setting, those who were in auditory-oral classrooms or mainstreamed (see Chapter 8) performed the best with their cochlear implants. Although this research is still ongoing and only the first few years of longitudinal data have been gathered and analyzed for these children, to date, these data indicate that about 50% of these profoundly hearing-impaired children who were implanted at an early age have achieved language and reading skills at or above their normal-hearing peers.

In the year 2000, there were about 30,000 cochlear implant wearers worldwide and about half of these were children (under the age of 18 years). In 2006, it was estimated that there were 100,000 cochlear implant recipients. Clearly, these devices are increasing in popularity and will most likely continue to do so as the technology continues to improve. Just as with hearing aids, the devices have continued to become physically smaller and less conspicuous while concurrently improving the signal-processing technology. Technologies that have proven to be somewhat successful with hearing aids, such as directional microphones to improve speech understanding in noise, are also being investigated with cochlear implants. One current issue under investigation by researchers is the relative benefit of bilateral cochlear implants, or the combination of an implant on one ear and a high-powered hearing aid on the other ear, over a single cochlear implant.

The importance of amplification or cochlear implantation to the hearing-impaired child cannot be overemphasized. The personal hearing aid or cochlear implant and other amplification devices are the primary link many of these children have to an auditory society. If these children are to develop speech and language in a manner somewhat similar to that of the normal-hearing child, everything possible must be done to capitalize on whatever residual hearing exists. Toward this end, the child receives amplification (usually binaural) or cochlear implantation (currently, usually monaural) soon after identification. The audiologist then offers periodic hearing evaluations and modifies the hearing aid fitting(s) or cochlear implant processor as more is learned about the child's hearing sensitivity.

DEVICE MANAGEMENT

The prosthetic device, whether a hearing aid, FM classroom device, or cochlear implant, is one of the most important aspects of rehabilitation for the majority of hearing-impaired individuals. It is essential that every precaution be taken to assure that the device is always in good working order.

For the vast majority of hearing-impaired individuals, the conventional electroacoustic hearing aid is the prosthetic device of choice. Care must be taken to avoid dropping the instrument or exposing the aid to severe environmental conditions, such as excessive moisture or heat. If dampness reaches the microphone or receiver, it can render the unit inoperable. It is also important to check the earmold or canal portion of the device periodically for blockage by cerumen and signs of wear from extended use, such as a cracked earmold or tubing. Perhaps the most common problem that interferes with adequate hearing-aid performance is the battery or battery compartment area. Old batteries that have lost their charge, inappropriate battery size, inadequate battery contact, and improper battery placement are all problems that can contribute to a nonworking hearing aid.

Consistent amplification for the young child with hearing impairment is essential. Yet numerous school surveys have revealed that approximately one-half of children's hearing aids do not perform satisfactorily. The most common problems seen among hearing-impaired children are weak batteries, inadequate earmolds, broken cords, bad receivers (sometimes the wrong receiver), and high distortion levels. Even the FM wireless systems are susceptible to faulty performance. Approximately 30% to 50% of these systems have been reported to perform unsatisfactorily in the classroom setting. The solution to inconsistent and inadequate amplification is the implementation of a daily hearing-aid check using a form like the one shown in Table 7.1. In addition, the school audiologist must conduct a periodic electroacoustic analysis of every child's hearing aid.

SUMMARY

In this chapter, we have reviewed and discussed the more pertinent aspects of amplification, cochlear implantation, and rehabilitation of hearing-impaired children and adults. It was noted that the hearing aid and the cochlear implant are the most important rehabilitative tools we have available to us for the management of the hearing-impaired. Numerous types of amplification systems, including personal hearing aids, assistive listening devices, and classroom systems, are available for the habilitation/rehabilitation of hearing-impaired individuals.

TABLE 7.1   Sample Monitoring Form for a Personal Hearing Aid Worn by a Hearing-Impaired Child

Student _____

Teacher _____ Aid make/model _____

School _____ Serial no. _____

Classroom _____

Electroacoustic check _____ Y _____ N

Date of inspection _____

Overall condition: ____ Satisfactory _____ Marginal ____ Unsatisfactory ____ Missing

Recommendations _____

_____

_____

Examiner _____

Problem Checklist

Item	Inspected?: Yes	No	Comments
Battery	_____	_____	_____
Battery compartment	_____	_____	_____
Microphone	_____	_____	_____
Power switch	_____	_____	_____
Gain control	_____	_____	_____
Telephone switch	_____	_____	_____
Tone control	_____	_____	_____
Amplifier	_____	_____	_____
Cord	_____	_____	_____
Receiver	_____	_____	_____
Earmold	_____	_____	_____
Clip/case	_____	_____	_____
Harness	_____	_____	_____
Other	_____	_____	_____

As-worn setting:

Volume control _____

Tone control _____

Receiver type _____

CHAPTER REVIEW QUESTIONS

1. Consider two 9-year-old children in a classroom, one of whom has a mild (35 dB HL) flat bilateral sensorineural hearing loss and the other who has a profound (90 dB HL) flat bilateral sensorineural hearing loss. Assume that the hearing loss was present and identified at birth in both children and that optimal early intervention focusing on an auditory-oral approach to rehabilitation followed the identification of hearing loss. What would be the auditory prosthetic device most likely used by each child? Why?

2. For each child in Question 1 above, would it be likely that supplemental auditory prosthetic devices would be used in the classroom? Address this separately for each child and indicate which device(s), if any, would be used by each child in the classroom.

3. Regardless of how you answered Question 1 above, assume for this question that both children have been fit with hearing aids and a two-thirds gain rule was used to set the gain of the hearing aids. How much gain in dB is needed at each frequency by each child? Assuming that this gain is achieved for each child and there is no limit to output, what would be the output of the hearing aids be for each child when a 60-dB-SPL input is provided to the hearing aid? For a 90-dB-SPL input? Would this cause any problems for the wearer and, if so, how might this be remedied?

SUGGESTED READINGS

Bess FH, Gravel JS, Tharpe AM. *Amplification for Children with Auditory Deficits.* Nashville: Bill Wilkerson Center Press; 1996.

Blamey PJ, Sarant JZ, Paatsch LE, et al. Relationships among speech perception, production, language, hearing loss, and age in children with impaired hearing. *J Speech Lang Hear Res.* 2001;44:264–285.

Byrne D. Theoretical prescriptive approaches to selecting the gain and frequency response of a hearing aid. *Monogr Contemp Audiol.* 1983;4:1–40.

Connor CM. Speech, vocabulary, and the education of children using cochlear implants. Oral or total communication? *J Speech Lang Hear Res.* 2000;43: 1185–1204.

Connor CM. Examining multiple sources of influence on the reading comprehension skills of children who use cochlear implants. *J Speech Lang Hear Res.* 2004;47:509–526.

Dillon H. *Hearing Aids.* New York: Thieme; 2001.

Geers AE, Moog JS. Predicting spoken language acquisition of profoundly hearing impaired children. *J Speech Hear Dis.* 1987;52:84–94.

Geers AE, Brenner C, Davidson L. Factors associated with development of speech perception skills in children implanted by age five. *Ear Hear.* 2003;24:24S–35S.

Geers AE, Nicholas JG, Sedey AL. Language skills of children with early cochlear implantation. *Ear Hear.* 2003;24:46S–58S.

Geers AE. Predictors of reading skill development in children with early cochlear implantation. *Ear Hear.* 2003;24:59S–68S.

Giolas TE, Owens E, Lamb SH, Schubert ED. Hearing performance inventory. *J Speech Hear Dis.* 1979;44:169–195.

Hawkins D, Yacullo W. The signal-to-noise ratio advantage of binaural hearing aids and directional microphones under different levels of reverberation. *J Speech Hearing Dis.* 1984;49:278–286.

High WS, Fairbanks G, Glorig A. Scale for self-assessment of hearing handicap. *J Speech Hear Dis.* 1964;17:321–327.

Katz J. *Handbook of Clinical Audiology.* 6th ed. Baltimore: Lippincott Williams & Wilkins, in press.

Moeller MP, Brunt MA. Management of preschool hearing-impaired children: A cognitive-linguistic approach. In Bess FH, ed. *Hearing Impairment in Children.* Parkton, MD: York Press; 1988.

Moeller MP, Carney AE. Assessment and intervention with preschool hearing-impaired children. In Alpiner JG, McCarthy PA, eds. *Rehabilitative Audiology: Children and Adults.* 2nd ed. Baltimore: Williams & Wilkins; 1993.

Mueller HG, Grimes A. Amplification systems for the hearing impaired. In Alpiner JF, McCarthy PA, eds. *Rehabilitative Audiology: Children and Adults.* Baltimore: Williams & Wilkins; 1987.

Mueller HG, Grimes MA. Hearing aid selection and assessment. In: Alpiner JG, McCarthy PA, eds. *Rehabilitative Audiology: Children and Adults.* 2nd ed. Baltimore: Williams & Wilkins; 1993.

Mueller HG, Hawkins DB, Northern JL. *Probe Microphone Measurements: Hearing Aid Selection and Assessment.* San Diego: Singular; 1992.

Mueller HG, Johnson EE, Carter AS. Hearing Aids and Assistive Devices. In Schow RL, Nerbonne MA, eds. Introduction to Audiologic Rehabilitation. 5th ed. Boston: Allyn and Bacon; 2007.

Northern JL, Downs MP. *Hearing in Children.* 5th Ed. Baltimore: Lippincott Williams & Wilkins; 2002.

Pascoe DP. *Hearing Aids. Who Needs Them?* St. Louis: Big Bend Books; 1991.

Ricketts TA, Tharpe AM, DeChicchis AR, Bess FH. Amplification selection for children with hearing impairment. In Bluestone CD, Alper CM, Arjmand EM, et al., eds. *Pediatric Otolaryngology.* 4th ed. Philadelphia: Harcourt Health Sciences; 2001.

Sanders DA. *Management of Hearing Handicap: Infants to Elderly.* 4th ed. Englewood Cliffs, NJ: Prentice Hall; 1999.

Schow, RL, Nerbonne, MA. *Introduction to Audiologic Rehabilitation*. 5th ed. Boston: Pearson Education; 2007.

Seewald RC. *A Sound Foundation Through Early Amplification*. Chicago: Phonak; 2000.

Seewald RC, Gravel JS. *A Sound Foundation Through Early Amplification, 2001*. Chicago: Phonak; 2002.

Skinner MW. *Hearing Aid Evaluation*. Englewood Cliffs, NJ: Prentice-Hall; 1988.

Studebaker GA, Bess FH. The Vanderbilt Hearing Aid Report. *Monogr Contemp Audiol*. 1982.

Studebaker GA, Bess FH, Beck LB. *The Vanderbilt Hearing Aid Report II*. Parkton, MD: York Press; 1991.

The Pediatric Work Group of the Conference on Amplification for Children with Auditory Deficits. Amplification for infants and children with hearing loss. *Am J Audiol*. 1996;5:53–68.

CHAPTER 8

Rehabilitation and Habilitation for Individuals with Impaired Hearing

- To appreciate the value of and need for aural rehabilitation or habilitation for individuals with impaired hearing;
- To recognize the differences in the details of the aural rehabilitation process for children versus adults, as well as children who experience impaired hearing before versus after the acquisition of spoken language; and
- To understand the elements of the aural rehabilitation process, including selection, fitting, and maintenance of the auditory prosthetic device, auditory training, speechreading, instruction in effective communication and communication strategies, and counseling.

KEY TERMS AND DEFINITIONS

- **Auditory-oral communication:** The education and rehabilitation of the person with impaired hearing is entirely based on auditory and oral communication. Training focuses on optimal use of hearing and speech for communication.
- **Total communication:** A manual communication system that is taught to supplement, to varying degrees, the auditory-oral communication of the person with impaired hearing.
- **Auditory training:** A variety of sound-based training programs focusing on individual speech sounds, words, or sentences and designed to enhance the perception and understanding of speech by persons with impaired hearing.
- **Speechreading:** Also often referred to as "lipreading," this is the process whereby the listener uses the visible facial gestures of the talker (not just the talker's lips) during speech production to better understand the spoken message.

As noted, breaks in the communication chain resulting from conductive pathologies are typically remedied via medical intervention, with some exceptions. For those with damage to the sensory structures in the cochlea, however, the damage is permanent and currently not subject to medical remediation. Alternative approaches to repairing the break in the communication chain are required.

Probably the most significant problem experienced by the adult with hearing loss is difficulty understanding speech, especially against a background of noise. Individuals with severe or profound sensorineural hearing loss also have trouble hearing speech in quiet settings and hearing their own speech. The inability to monitor their own speech typically results in speech production problems as well, making the overall communication process even more difficult. The intent of rehabilitation for the hearing-impaired adult is to restore as much speech-comprehension and speech-production ability as possible. That is, the goal is to circumvent any breaks in the communication chain resulting from an auditory impairment and restore normal or near-normal communication.

For the child with congenital hearing impairment, however, the problem is more complicated because the symbols of our language system have not yet been learned. Vocabulary is being acquired and the rules of the child's grammar are being formed. As noted previously, vocabulary and syntax develop naturally in the typically developing child through repeated exposures to spoken language. For the young child with impaired hearing, the emphasis is on helping the child to acquire this complex language system and to use language appropriately so that communication skills might be gained. The focus is more on habilitation than on rehabilitation. In other words, the objective is not to restore a skill that once existed, but to help the child develop a new skill, the ability to communicate orally and auditorily.

As noted in Chapter 7, the central core of any rehabilitation/habilitation program is the use of a prosthetic device that compensates for the individual's hearing loss. The most common such device is the hearing aid, but, in more severe impairments, the cochlear implant, a device that bypasses the damaged cochlea and stimulates the auditory nerve fibers electrically, is becoming more commonplace. (See Chapter 7 for more details.) Typically, the fitting of the device is the first step in the intervention-phase of an aural rehabilitation program. This chapter focuses on the provision of treatment that follows the fitting of the prosthetic device. The treatment differs considerably for children and adults. As a result, each is the focus of a separate section of this chapter.

REHABILITATION OF THE CHILD WITH HEARING IMPAIRMENT

Management of the child with hearing impairment is a monumental challenge to the clinical audiologist. In learning to understand the spoken language of others and to speak it, there is no adequate substitute for an intact auditory system. Without normal or near-normal hearing, it is extremely difficult to acquire an adequate oral communication system. Because so much of the language-learning process occurs within the first few years of life, there has been considerable emphasis on early identification and intervention for young hearing-impaired children. The various approaches to early identification were outlined in Chapter 6 and will not be restated here. For the most part, however, the earlier one can identify the hearing loss, preferably during the first several months of life, the sooner intervention can begin and the better the chances for a favorable outcome. Generally speaking, hearing-impaired children who exhibit the best spoken language and show the most satisfactory progress in school are those who have had the benefit of early identification and intervention. Early intervention is essential to the successful development of speech and language. The intervention must include adequate parent-infant management, wearable amplification or cochlear implants, speech and language training, and development of perceptual and cognitive skills, including listening skills.

Choosing the Appropriate Communication Mode

An important issue facing audiologists, teachers, and school officials is determining which educational approach is most appropriate for a given hearing-impaired child. Presently, two primary modes of instruction are recommended in the educational system: **auditory-oral communication** and **total communication**. The auditory-oral approach places emphasis entirely on the auditory system for developing receptive and expressive forms of communication, whereas total communication emphasizes a combination of audition, vision, finger spelling, and signs for achieving the same goal. As noted in Chapter 1, the emphasis in this is on the development of auditory-oral communication. Recent research is somewhat equivocal regarding the superiority of one approach over the other, especially in various areas of language abilities and when giving the child the opportunity to be assessed using oral only or oral plus sign language. Not surprisingly, however, this same research reveals superior performance of children in auditory-oral environments when either their speech perception abilities or the clarity of their own speech productions have been evaluated.

Let us now review some of the appropriate management strategies for hearing-impaired children. The approaches to be discussed can accommodate either an auditory-oral or a total communication emphasis.

Parent-Infant Management

The first 3 years of life are critical to a child's general development, especially with respect to communication, and the parents of young handicapped children often lack the skills necessary to optimize family-infant interactions, which could facilitate the child's communication development. Awareness of this situation has led to parent-infant intervention programs. In addition to espousing early identification and intervention, most parent-oriented programs include family support for parents and members of the child's extended family. Information sharing or exchange, demonstration teaching (in which the family explores a variety of strategies to assist the child in achieving communication), and educational advocacy for the parents are also frequently included. The latter entails helping the parents to become effective consumers of services and knowledgeable child advocates.

An important component of a parent-infant curriculum is audiologic management and amplification or cochlear implantation. Here the emphasis is on helping the child to develop his or her auditory potential. Emphasis is placed on further clarification of the nature of the hearing loss, selection of amplification, and the development of full-time hearing aid use. Teaching parents the importance of care and maintenance of hearing aids is also an important dimension.

Another element of effective parent-infant management is **auditory training**, an organized sequential approach to the development of listening skills. Here, the emphasis is on developing a program of auditory training experiences that will guide the parents through a developmental sequence for their child that parallels the development of auditory perceptual skills in the normal-hearing infant. The hierarchy of skills can be divided into the following levels:

1. Auditory perception of both environmental sounds and the human voice
2. Awareness of environmental sounds and the human voice as conveyors of information and association of sounds with their physical sources
3. Development of an auditory-vocal feedback mechanism in which the child monitors his or her own speech
4. Comprehension of meaning in syllables, words, phrases, and sentences
5. Increasing verbal comprehension and the emergence of auditory memory and sequencing skills

Another important component of parent-infant management is vocal play strategies for speech habilitation. The initiation and maintenance of vocal behavior is a major area of the early-intervention program that is critical to young children. Full-time use of hearing aids or cochlear implants is important so that the hearing-impaired child can hear his or her own speech as well as the speech of others. The use of an auditory program to enhance the use of the auditory feedback mechanism is also important. Further, parents are taught to use vocal play interaction techniques that are necessary for the development of prelinguistic speech skills. Parents must also learn to develop strategies that facilitate social and communicative turn-taking.

Finally, there are the verbal interaction techniques of language programming. At this point, the focus is on teaching the parent communicative interaction styles, particularly verbal interaction patterns, which enhance the child's acquisition of language. Linguistic development is maximized by training parents to incorporate the principles of adult-child interaction patterns that are reported to occur during the language acquisition of normal children.

Language: Characteristics, Assessment, and Training

As noted in the discussion of the communication chain in Chapter 1, language may be defined as a systematic code used to represent the concepts that designate experience and to facilitate social interaction. Oral language is the primary means by which humans communicate with one another. Although a comprehensive review of language is beyond the scope of this book, a general knowledge of the dimensions of language is important to the understanding of management issues. Most would agree that there are three components of language: form, content, and use. The form of language pertains to the elements of language and the rules for combining those elements. The three aspects of language form include phonology (the sounds or phonemes of the language), syntax (word order rules), and morphology (the internal structure of words). In learning phonology, children acquire the rules for how sounds can be sequenced to formulate words. For example, in English, the /mp/ sequence of phonemes can appear at the end of a word (e.g., jump), but not at the beginning of a word. In learning syntax, children acquire the rules for how words are combined to form grammatical sentences. For example, when forming a question, a subject-noun and an auxiliary ("He is . . .") can be reversed (e.g., "Is he eating cookies?"), but a subject-noun and main verb ("He eats . . .") cannot be inverted (e.g., ungrammatical: "Eats he cookies?"). Lastly, in learning morphology, children acquire the rules for how inflections are added to words (e.g., the plural of cookie is cookies). To learn language, children must process language input (e.g., the talk of their caregiver) and hypothesize the rules to formulate grammatical sentences.

The second component of language is content, also referred to as semantics. Children must learn the meaning of individual words, as well as the meaning of particular phrases (e.g., "raining cats and dogs").

The final component of language is pragmatics, or the ability to use language to communicate effectively; that is, how to engage in conversation and how to use language to meet a variety of goals (e.g., seek information, answer questions). The development of language is an extremely complex process, involving the acquisition of skill in each component of language.

Given what we have discussed about language, it is not surprising to learn that children with hearing loss experience great difficulty in learning language through speech. This difficulty increases with increasing hearing loss. Most research dealing with the language characteristics of children with hearing loss has focused on the "form" component, because errors in form (phonemes, morphemes, and syntax) are easier to quantify. In addition, the acquisition of form may be more challenging than the acquisition of content and use. Nevertheless, it is important to realize that researchers have documented language learning difficulties in all aspects of language, form, content, and use for children with hearing loss.

Many commercially available instruments are designed to assist the clinician in the ongoing evaluation of a child's language development. Although formal language tests explore a wide range of language skills, for the most part, they do not adequately evaluate a child's ability to use language in day-to-day situations. Hence, clinicians always need to explore informal nonstandardized tasks to obtain information in areas not covered by the standard diagnostic tools. Language sampling can be an invaluable tool in determining the extent to which hearing loss is affecting the development and the interaction of content, form, and use in the child's language system as the child engages in authentic communication.

A number of approaches have been used in language intervention, most of which have focused on the syntactic forms of language. These approaches can be classified as either analytic or natural methods for teaching language. Analytic methods have concentrated on the form of a child's language, and most techniques categorize the various parts of speech grammatically. These approaches are also characterized by extensive drills and exercises. An example of the analytical method is the Fitzgerald key, which emphasizes the analysis of relationships among discrete units through the visual aid of written language. Students classify words from a sentence as to whether they belong in a "who," "what," or "where" category. The natural approach, sometimes referred to as the experiential method, holds that language is learned through experiences, not systematic drills and exercises. This content/unit approach emphasizes identifying areas of interest for the child that then serve as the basis for teaching vocabulary in meaningful contexts and practicing spoken and, later, written language.

More recently, language-intervention approaches have begun to consider modern language theory and to develop strategies that attempt to integrate syntactic, pragmatic, and semantic levels. The reader interested in learning more about language intervention techniques based on current theory for individuals with hearing loss can consult the suggested readings at the end of this chapter.

Speech Production: Characteristics, Assessment, and Training

It was noted earlier that significant hearing losses make it difficult not only to understand speech, but also to produce speech. The auditory feedback portion of the communication chain is impaired. Nevertheless, it is the general consensus that many hearing-impaired children, even those with profound losses, can develop speech skills. This is especially true for profoundly impaired children who received early intervention using cochlear implants and were educated in using an auditory-oral approach. Hearing-impaired children manifest a variety of speech production errors categorized as either segmental (i.e., phonemic and phonetic) or suprasegmental (i.e., related to intonation and prosody). The most common segmental errors include the omission of word-final sounds and substitution errors for both consonants and vowels. Suprasegmental errors include inadequate timing, which results in very slow, labored speech, and poor control of the fundamental frequency, which causes abnormal pitch and distorted intonation. Predictably, as the frequency of errors increases, overall intelligibility decreases and the communication chain is increasingly ineffective.

Assessment of speech production is not as easy as one might predict because many of the tools were designed for normal-hearing children. The evaluation of segmental errors is usually conducted with commonly available picture identification tests. Because most of these tests do not consider the unavoidable problems of testing the child with hearing impairment, it is not unusual for the clinician to develop informal tests that will focus on specific segmental errors frequently seen in this population. Assessment of overall intelligibility of conversational speech is also important for the planning of an intervention program. Some clinicians record spontaneous speech samples, which are then judged by a group of listeners to evaluate a child's intelligibility.

Perhaps the most popular method for teaching speech to the hearing-impaired child is an approach advocated by Daniel Ling. Very briefly, this method focuses on using the child's residual hearing to monitor speech production, as well as to understand the speech of others. The approach to speech acquisition attempts to duplicate the process that normal-hearing children experience. The teaching of speech is carried out primarily at the phonetic and phonologic levels, with emphasis on the phonetic domain. At the phonetic level, there is emphasis on nonsense syllable drills (i.e., /ta, ta, ta/ or /ti, ta, to/). Several stages are proposed in which target behaviors are established using criterion-referenced skills. A child must complete each phase satisfactorily before moving on to the next level. These stages include undifferentiated vocalizations; suprasegmental voice patterns; a range of distinctly different vowel sounds; consonants contrasted in manner of production; consonants contrasted in manner and place of production; consonants contrasted in manner, place, and voicing; and consonant blends. The following additional strategies have been suggested to supplement the Ling approach:

1. Production by imitation: the child produces the target sound using auditory clues only;
2. Production on demand: the child produces the target sound from visual cues;
3. Discrimination: the child selects the speech pattern from a closed set of alternative speech patterns produced by the clinician or model; and
4. Self-evaluation: the child evaluates his or her own speech production.

REHABILITATION OF THE ADULT WITH IMPAIRED HEARING

The rehabilitation techniques used with the hearing-impaired adult are quite different from the approaches used with children. There are similarities, however. The individual must receive a careful assessment to determine the nature and extent of the problem, amplification plays a major role in the rehabilitation process, and the techniques and strategies used in rehabilitation are determined by the information elicited in the assessment phase. Although cochlear implants can be used by adults with profoundly impaired hearing, the overwhelming majority of adults with hearing impairment have losses that are milder and most appropriately addressed through hearing aids.

Assessment Issues

In the introduction to this chapter, we talked about the importance of the assessment phase and how it is used to establish a rehabilitative program. The assessment phase typically consists of a comprehensive case history, pure-tone audiometry, immittance measurements, speech-recognition tests, a communication-specific self-assessment questionnaire, and, occasionally, a measure of speechreading ability. Because we have already reviewed in some detail the basic assessment battery (case history, pure-tone audiometry, immittance measurements, and speech recognition), we will focus here on questionnaires and speechreading skills in the planning of rehabilitation programs.

Assessment with Communication Scales

Communication scales need to be a part of every assessment approach. These scales usually assess how the hearing impairment affects everyday living, for example, the way in which the hearing deficit affects psychosocial, emotional, or vocational performance. Such information can be of value in determining the need for and probable success of amplification, irrespective of the degree of hearing loss and the specific areas in which the rehabilitation should occur. Most scales have focused on communication-specific skills. Examples of questions that could be included in such a scale are: "Do you have difficulty hearing when someone speaks in a whisper?" and "Does a hearing problem cause you difficulty when listening to TV or radio?"

The answers to such questions illuminate listening problems. Once the areas of difficulty have been identified, possible solutions can be considered. For example, if the individual reports difficulty only when listening to a television or radio, an assistive listening device might be considered. If, on the other hand, a patient reports difficulty in a variety of listening situations and notes a tendency to withdraw from social activities because of the hearing loss, the individual would be a good candidate for a personal hearing aid. Counseling for this patient and the patient's relatives might also be indicated. Furthermore, the clinician may wish to develop techniques for improving speechreading and auditory training skills in situations that present listening difficulty. Numerous communication scales are available for use.

Management Strategies with the Hearing-Impaired Adult

Importance of Counseling

Counseling should be a central focus of any management strategy for the adult with hearing loss. In fact, the hearing-impaired adult should receive counseling both before and after the provision of a hearing aid. Counseling is a vital part of the assessment phase because it is during this phase that information about the patient's communication problems is determined. The first component of the counseling process is to explain to the patient, in lay terms, the nature and extent of the hearing loss. If the audiologist believes that the patient can benefit from amplification, counseling is needed to discuss with the patient the value of a hearing aid and what can be expected from it. Possible modification of the patient's motivation and attitudes may also be appropriate at this juncture. The audiologist will have information from the assessment data on the patient's feelings about wearing a hearing aid. Often the patient has no real interest in a hearing aid but is simply responding to the will of a spouse or "significant other." Others have received misleading information about hearing aids from friends or from advertisements. Some patients are concerned about whether the hearing aid will show because of the stigma commonly associated with deafness in the United States (Vignette 8.1). Under such circumstances, the objective of the audiologist is to help the hearing-impaired individual realize that many of the fears or concerns about hearing loss or hearing aids are unwarranted. The individual should be counseled that the use of amplification can help in a variety of listening situations.

Counseling is also sometimes appropriate for relatives and friends who have developed erroneous impressions about hearing loss and amplification. For example, a patient with a high-frequency sensorineural hearing loss will typically experience difficulty in understanding speech. Relatives and friends sometimes interpret this difficulty as a sign of senility, inattention, or even stupidity. It is helpful for the audiologist to counsel relatives and friends about the nature and extent of hearing loss as well as the psychosocial complications associated with a hearing deficit. Reviewing such information with loved ones helps them to understand better and to be more tolerant of the listening difficulties caused by a significant hearing impairment. The audiologist may also choose to offer suggestions for enhancing communication. The significant other can be counseled in the use of deliberate, unhurried speech, good illumination of the speaker's face, and care to ensure that the lips are clearly visible.

Once the hearing aid has been purchased, or just before a purchase, the patient is counseled about the use and care of a hearing aid. The audiologist reviews the manipulation of the various controls, the function of the battery compartment, troubleshooting techniques in case of malfunction, the proper care of the earmold or shell, and the warranty of the hearing aid. A potential difficulty is that patients often have unrealistic expectations for a hearing aid, especially in the initial stages of use. The audiologist must take care to advise the hearing-impaired patient about the limitations of amplification and to help the individual adjust to very difficult listening situations, such as competing speech or the presence of a competing background noise. Finally, some patients will need special help in the manipulation of hearing aid controls. This is a common problem among the elderly.

Throughout the entire rehabilitation cycle, counseling is seen as a continuing process. The audiologist spends time listening, advising, and reacting to the needs and concerns of the hearing-impaired individual.

VIGNETTE 8.1   FURTHER DISCUSSION

THE HEARING AID EFFECT

Examine the two top pictures. How would you rate the person on the left on a continuum from bright to dull? From smart to dumb? From pretty to ugly? How about the person on the right at the top?

Now, examine the bottom two pictures. How would you rate these two individuals on the same continua listed above?

Notice that the two people pictured in the top set of "photographs" are the same as the two in the bottom set, but the one wearing the hearing aid has changed. When researchers have had large groups of subjects rate their impressions of real photographs similar to these drawings along continua similar to those listed above and have counterbalanced the design so that each person is pictured wearing a hearing aid by the conclusion of the testing, the results indicate that the presence of a hearing aid on the individual in the photo leads to lower ratings on many continua. This negative image associated with the wearing of a hearing aid is called "the hearing aid effect." It has been documented in adults and children alike and is part of the stigma hearing aid wearers must overcome.

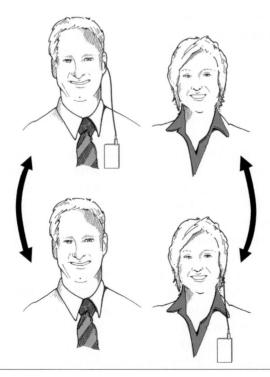

Instruction for Speechreading and Auditory Training

The two primary training aspects of aural rehabilitation for the adult are speechreading and auditory training. Speechreading refers to the ability of a person, any person, to use vision as a supplement to audition when communicating. All persons, regardless of the degree of impairment, can benefit from visual cues. At one time, speechreading was referred to simply as "lipreading." The change in label to "speechreading" has come about in recognition of the fact that more than just the talker's lips provide important visual cues to understanding speech.

Speechreading should be viewed not as a replacement for auditory coding of speech, but as an important supplement. With visual information alone, approximately 40% to 50% of a "spoken" message typically can be understood by the average person (the actual level of performance varies depending on a wide variety of factors including the context of the message and numerous factors regarding the visibility of the talker). However, for a given set of conditions, individuals vary widely in this ability.

Acquisition of speechreading skills can take hours of training. There are two basic approaches to speechreading training: analytic and synthetic. Analytic methods begin with training on individual speech sounds and progress to words, phrases, sentences, and continuous discourse, in sequence. The synthetic approach begins training at the phrase or sentence level. The synthetic approach seems to be the one more widely used by audiologists. Training usually begins with simple, commonly encountered questions such as, "What is your name?" or "What time is it?" It then progresses to less frequently encountered statements and continuous discourse.

Auditory training refers to teaching the individual with hearing loss to use his or her hearing as well as possible. The approaches pursued vary with the onset of the hearing loss. Typically, a hierarchy of skills is developed at the phoneme and word level, beginning with detection of the sound or word (can the patient hear anything when the sound is spoken?). The next goal is discrimination of the targeted sound or word (is it the same or different from some other sounds or words?), followed by the development of skills in the identification of the sound or word (which one of several words or sounds was it?). The final goal is often to develop proficiency in the open-set recognition of the speech sound or word (what sound or word was it?). Auditory training is encouraged for all individuals wearing a hearing aid for the first time. It takes time and training to learn to understand speech with a hearing aid. Many individuals with hearing loss have never heard speech or have heard it through the distortion of the hearing loss—in many cases, for a period of several years—before seeking assistance. Fitting the hearing aid or other rehabilitative device will not bring about an instant restoration of normal function. Recent research indicates that at least 3 to 6 months may be required for many hearing-aid wearers to attain maximum levels of speech-communication performance with their hearing aids. In fact, many patients will probably never perform *completely* as well as a normal-hearing person does, especially under adverse listening conditions all too commonly encountered in everyday communication situations. With continued training, however, they can come much closer to achieving this objective. Auditory training is designed to maximize the use of residual hearing, whereas speechreading is meant to supplement the reduced information received through the auditory system. Extensive training in both areas can result in very effective use of the rehabilitative device chosen for the patient.

LISTENING TRAINING, SPEECH CONSERVATION, AND SPEECH TRACKING

Another role of the audiologist is to help the hearing-impaired patient develop or maintain good listening skills and to assist the patient in maintaining good speech production skills. Listening training refers to helping the patient to attend better to the spoken message. Some people simply have poor listening skills, and this problem is exacerbated in the presence of a hearing loss. The emphasis in listening training is on teaching the impaired listener to be alert, attentive, and ready to receive the spoken message. Training should focus on eliminating or avoiding distractions, learning to focus on the speaker's main points, attending to nonverbal information, keeping visual contact with the speaker, and mentally preparing oneself to listen to the speaker.

As hearing loss increases, it becomes more difficult for an individual to monitor his or her own speech production. This inability results in faulty speech characterized by poor vocal quality, nasality, segmental errors, and suprasegmental errors. Under such conditions, learning the effective use of kinesthetic (sensation of movement) cues is essential for creating an awareness of the segmental elements of speech. The patient must become physically aware of the kinesthetic qualities of each phonetic element in speech. Auditory training and speechreading can also help in preserving the perception of subtle nuances in the speech message. Techniques for developing an awareness of the rhythm, quality, intonation, and loudness of one's own speech are needed by the hearing impaired. Finally, the importance of listening is critical to this population, and the enhancement of listening skills should be part of any speech-conservation program.

Speech tracking refers to a procedure in which a reader presents connected speech and a listener repeats the message, word-for-word or syllable–for-syllable. Both the speaker and the listener participate in the procedure, with the impaired listener attempting to immediately imitate the speaker. The technique has great face validity because the material approximates normal communication more closely than single words do. Tracking ability is measured in terms of the number of words tracked per minute. Rate of speech tracking improves with rehabilitative training (speechreading and/or auditory training) and with the use of amplification or alternative rehabilitation devices. Speech tracking can be used as a tool in aural rehabilitation, especially for measuring the effects of rehabilitation or training.

SPECIAL CONSIDERATIONS FOR THE HEARING-IMPAIRED ELDERLY

We have noted on several occasions throughout this text that a large number of elderly people exhibit significant hearing impairments. Typically, the hearing impairment in the aged is a mild-to-moderate, bilateral, high-frequency sensorineural hearing loss with associated difficulty in understanding conversational speech (Chapter 3). The loss usually begins around 50 years of age and progresses with each succeeding decade. In addition, speech understanding difficulties become greater when the listening task is made more difficult. Such hearing loss adversely affects both the functional health status and the psychosocial well-being of the impaired individual. It is generally thought that hearing loss can produce withdrawal, poor self-concept, depression, frustration, irritability, senility, isolation, and loneliness.

Despite the high prevalence of hearing loss among the elderly and the accepted psychosocial complications, the hearing-impaired elderly are not usually referred for audiologic intervention. Frequently, they are not considered candidates for amplification until they reach advanced old age. The reasons for this are not clear. Some elderly persons believe that their deafness is simply another unavoidable aspect of the aging process. This feeling lessens the person's felt need to seek rehabilitation or the ability to justify it. This belief, combined with an inadequate knowledge and low expectations of rehabilitative measures, seems to discourage these individuals from seeking assistance. Even those who do seek assistance often fail to use their hearing aids to the fullest. In fact, some stop using their amplification systems soon after purchase.

The special problems of the hearing-impaired elderly require that the audiologist educate physicians and laypersons about the benefits of hearing aids. Audiologists must also recognize the special needs of this population. For example, during the assessment phase, one must determine whether there are any limitations in upper body movement or if arthritis exists. These conditions can interfere with an individual's ability to reach, grasp, or manipulate a hearing aid. Such information is most helpful in deciding on the type of hearing aid to be recommended. For example, a small in-the-canal hearing aid with microcontrols would be inappropriate for an individual who has arthritis affecting the hands and arms. Another important consideration in the assessment phase is the visual acuity of the patient. Like hearing, vision declines with increasing age. Because visual acuity is important for receiving auditory-visual information, it is prudent for the audiologist to assess the visual abilities of an elderly patient. This can be done simply by posing questions about visual status to the hearing-impaired person. Examples of such questions might include:

1. Do you have problems with your vision? If so, what kind?
2. Do you wear eyeglasses? Do they help you to see?
3. Are you able to see my mouth clearly?

Some audiologists actually test for far-visual acuity using the well-known Snellen eye chart.

A check of mental status is also appropriate for the elderly population. Many elderly individuals exhibit declines in cognitive function that would reduce the likelihood of successful use of a hearing aid. Formal tests are available to assess mental status. In lieu of these, however, the audiologist can simply pose questions that will offer information about the patient's cognitive functioning (i.e., memory, general knowledge, orientation). If there are problems with mental status, the audiologist will need to work closely with a significant other to assure appropriate use and care of the hearing aid.

Other factors that need to be considered before amplification is recommended to an elderly person include motivation, family support, financial resources, and lifestyle. Special attention is also important for the elderly during the hearing aid orientation program. Greater care is required to explain the various components of a hearing aid. Furthermore, the audiologist should schedule elderly patients for periodic follow-up visits to monitor the patients' progress and to review questions and concerns that they may have about their amplification devices. When considering amplification for this group, one must recognize that they could benefit from many of the assistive listening devices described earlier in this chapter. Many of the problems experienced by this group involve use of the telephone, watching television, and understanding speech in group situations, such as church or public auditoriums.

To summarize, the hearing-impaired elderly have unique problems and concerns that require the special consideration of the clinician throughout the rehabilitation process. If the clinician attends to these needs and concerns, there is a far greater probability that use of a hearing aid will be successful.

SUMMARY

In this chapter, we have reviewed the treatment provided to children and adults with impaired hearing, after the prosthetic device has been fitted. Although the details differ considerably between various approaches and their application to children or adults, the end result is the same: restoration of the function of the normally functioning communication chain. Given that the hearing loss is associated with loss of sensory receptors, whether treated using a hearing aid or a cochlear implant, treatment is required after the fitting of the prosthetic device to optimize the benefits received.

CHAPTER REVIEW QUESTIONS

1. Consider two children with severe bilateral flat sensorineural hearing loss who are otherwise identical, except for the age at which the hearing loss occurred. One child developed the hearing loss at 4 years of age, whereas the hearing loss was present at birth in the other. Assume that the hearing loss was not detected until each child entered school at an age of 5 years. What would you anticipate as likely differences in the communication abilities of these two children when assessed by the clinician at the school?

2. How could the differences observed in the communication skills of the two 5-year-old children with severe hearing loss in Question 1 have been minimized or eliminated?

3. Older adults purchase two-thirds of the hearing aids sold in the United States, yet a majority of those who have purchased hearing aids indicate that they are less than satisfied with them. What factors might contribute to this less than ideal satisfaction and what steps might be taken to improve satisfaction and benefit from their hearing aids in older adults?

SUGGESTED READINGS

Alpiner JG, Schow RL. Rehabilitative evaluation of hearing-impaired adults. In: Alpiner JG, McCarthy PA, eds. *Rehabilitative Audiology: Children and Adults.* 2nd ed. Baltimore: Williams & Wilkins; 1993.

Bess FH, Gravel JS. *Foundations of Pediatric Audiology: A Book of Readings.* San Diego, CA: Plural, 2006.

Bess FH, Gravel JS, Tharpe AM. *Amplification for Children with Auditory Deficits.* Nashville: Bill Wilkerson Center Press; 1996.

Bloom L, Lahey M. *Language Development and Language Disorders.* New York: John Wiley & Sons; 1978.

Clark JG, Martin FN. *Effective Counseling in Audiology: Perspectives and Practice.* Englewood Cliffs, NJ: Prentice Hall; 1994.

Fitzgerald MT, Bess FH. Parent/infant training for hearing-impaired children. *Monogr Contemp Audiol.* 1982;3:1–24.

Geers AE, Moog JS. Predicting spoken language acquisition of profoundly hearing impaired children. *J Speech Hear Dis.* 1987;52:84–94.

Giolas TE, Owens E, Lamb SH, Schubert ED. Hearing performance inventory. *J Speech Hear Dis.* 1979;44:169–195.

High WS, Fairbanks G, Glorig A. Scale for self-assessment of hearing handicap. *J Speech Hear Dis.* 1964;17:321–327.

Katz J. *Handbook of Clinical Audiology.* 6th ed. Baltimore: Lippincott Williams & Wilkins, in press.

Kretschmer RR, Kretschmer LW. Communication/language assessment of the hearing-impaired child. In Bess FH, ed. *Hearing Impairment in Children.* Parkton, MD: York Press; 1988.

Kurtzer-White E, Luterman D. *Early Childhood Deafness.* Baltimore: York Press; 2001.

Ling D. *Speech and the Hearing-Impaired Child: Theory and Practice.* Washington, DC: Alexander Graham Bell Association for the Deaf; 1976.

Mitchell, RE, Karchmer, MA: More students in more places. *Am Ann Deaf.* 2006;151:95–104.

Moeller MP, Brunt MA. Management of preschool hearing-impaired children: A cognitive-linguistic approach. In Bess FH, ed: *Hearing Impairment in Children.* Parkton, MD: York Press; 1988.

Moeller MP, Carney AE. Assessment and intervention with preschool hearing-impaired children. In: Alpiner JG, McCarthy PA, eds: *Rehabilitative Audiology: Children and Adults.* 2nd Ed. Baltimore: Williams & Wilkins; 1993.

Norlin PF, Van Tassell DJ. Linguistic skills of hearing-impaired children. *Monogr Contemp Audiol.* 1980;2:1–32.

Sanders DA. *Management of Hearing Handicap: Infants to Elderly.* 4th ed. Englewood Cliffs, NJ: Prentice Hall; 1999.

Schow, RL, Nerbonne, MA. *Introduction to Audiologic Rehabilitation.* 5th ed. Boston: Pearson Education; 2007.

Seewald RC, Gravel JS, eds: *A Sound Foundation Through Early Amplification,* 2001. Chicago: Phonak; 2002.

Glossary

A

American Academy of Audiology
AAA; professional organization for audiologists.

ABR
Auditory brainstem response; a series of five to seven waves in the electrical waveform that appear in the first 10 ms after the presentation of an auditory stimulus such as a click or a tone burst. The ABR is sensitive to dysfunction occurring from the auditory periphery to the upper auditory brainstem portions of the auditory central nervous system.

Acoustic immittance measurements
Clinical measurement of the impedance or admittance of the flow of sound energy through the middle ear.

Acoustic neuroma
A tumor that affects the eighth/auditory nerve.

Acoustic reflex
Reflexive contractions of the middle ear muscles caused by the presentation of a sound stimulus.

Acoustic reflex threshold
Lowest possible intensity needed to elicit a middle ear muscle contraction.

Acquired hearing loss
Hearing loss obtained sometime after birth.

Acute otitis media
Middle ear disease of rapid onset and rapid resolution; characterized by a reddish or yellowish bulging tympanic membrane, obliteration of ossicular

landmarks, and conductive hearing loss.

Admittance
Ease of flow of energy through a system; reciprocal of impedance.

Afferent
Term pertaining to conduction of electrical activity via nerve fibers from peripheral to central locations; ascending nerve fibers.

American Sign Language
ASL; sign language used in the United States. Differs from other forms of manual communication devised to make signs more like the English language.

American Speech-Language-Hearing Association
ASHA; professional organization for Audiologists and Speech-Language Pathologists.

Anomaly
A deviation from normal.

ANSI
American National Standards Institute; organization that develops standards for measuring devices (e.g., audiometers).

Apex
Term used to denote the top or near the top.

Apgar score
A common assessment tool for describing the amount of depression exhibited by the infant at birth. Apgar scores consist of five criteria: (a) heart rate, (b) respiratory rate, (c) muscle tone, (d) response to stimulation, and (e) color. The highest possible score is 10.

Articulators
Anatomical structures, such as the lips, tongue and velum (soft palate), which are positioned in various ways by a talker to produce speech sounds.

Assistive listening device
A wide assortment of electronic devices designed as either alternatives to or supplements of other auditory prosthetic devices. Depending on the severity of the hearing loss, common assistive listening devices include wireless systems designed for use while watching television, systems to use while using the telephone, and the use of visual stimulation (e.g., flashing lights) for doorbells, alarm clocks, or other alerting devices.

Atresia
Absence or closure of a normal body opening; in hearing, it most often refers to the ear canal.

Audiogram
Graphic representation of a person's hearing. Sound level (in dB) is plotted on the ordinate and frequency is shown on the abscissa.

Audioscope
Hand-held otoscope with a built in audiometer.

Auditory central nervous system
Comprised of the ascending and descending auditory pathways and centers in the brainstem and cortex.

Auditory cortex
Auditory area of the cerebral cortex located primarily in the region of the temporal lobe.

Auditory-oral approach
Method used to teach children with significant hearing loss speech and language; emphasis is on hearing and speechreading with no manual communication.

Auditory periphery
Comprised of the outer ear, middle ear, and inner ear, ending at the nerve fibers exiting the inner ear.

Auditory-verbal approach Method used to teach children with significant hearing loss speech and language; emphasis is on listening and understanding the spoken message via the auditory system with no emphasis on vision for receiving information.

Auditory training A variety of sound-based training programs focusing on individual speech sounds, words or sentences and designed to enhance the perception and understanding of speech by persons with impaired hearing.

A-weighted scale A filtering network on the sound level meter that filters the low frequencies and approximates the response characteristics of the human ear.

B

Basal
Term used to denote near the end or base.

Basilar membrane
Membrane in the cochlear duct that supports the organ of Corti.

BC
Bone conduction; transmission of sound to the inner ear via the skull.

Bilateral
Term used to denote both sides.

Bilirubin
A red bile pigment, sometimes found in urine, which is present in the blood tissues during jaundice.

Binaural
Pertaining to both ears.

BOA
Behavioral observation audiometry; evaluation of a child's hearing via observation of responses (e.g., head turn) to sound.

Broadband (white) noise
An acoustic signal that contains energy of equal spectral density (intensity) at all frequencies.

BTE
Behind the ear.

C

Calibrate
To set the parameters of an instrument such as an audiometer to an accepted standard (e.g., ANSI).

CANS
Central auditory nervous system.

Carhart
Father of the profession of audiology.

Cholesteatoma
Accumulation of debris developed from perforations of the eardrum; sometimes referred to as a pseudo-like tumor.

Chromosome
One of several small rod-shaped bodies, easily stained, that appear in the nucleus of a cell at the time of cell division; they contain the genes, or hereditary factors, and are constant in number in each species.

Cilium (plural: cilia)
Minute, hair-like structures of sensory cells (inner and outer hair cells) in the cochlea.

Classroom amplification system
An electroacoustic system typically making use of a detached microphone worn by the teacher with the microphone's output sent to personal amplification units worn by members of the class who have impaired hearing.

Cochlea
Auditory portion of the inner ear; sensory organ for hearing.

Cochlear Implant
An electronic device that is surgically implanted under the skin behind the ear with electrodes (wires) extending through the middle ear and inserting into the fluid-filled cochlea. The normal transducer function of the inner ear is bypassed and the nerve fibers exiting the cochlea are stimulated directly by electrical current. These devices currently are reserved for use by individuals with severe or profound amounts of hearing loss who demonstrate little benefit from conventional hearing aids.

Collapsed canal
A canal that collapses as the result of pressure caused by earphone placement.

COM
Chronic otitis media. Otitis media that is slow in its onset, tends to be persistent, and often can produce other complications. The most common symptoms are hearing loss, perforation of the tympanic membrane, and fluid discharge.

Communication Chain
The sequence of events from the initiation of a thought, idea or emotion to be communicated by the sender through the reception and interpretation of that message by the receiver. For humans, the message is typically communicated acoustically via speech.

Compression
Technique used to decrease or limit the wide range of sounds in our everyday world to match more closely the dynamic range of listeners with hearing loss.

Computed tomography (CT)
Radiography in which a three dimensional image of a body structure is constructed by computer from a series of cross-sectional images.

Concha
Depression or bowl-shaped area of the auricle; serves to collect and direct sound to the external auditory meatus.

Congenital
Before birth; usually before the 28th week of gestation.

Contralateral
Pertaining to the opposite side.

Cortex
The outer layer of an organ, such as the cerebrum or cerebellum.

Cytomegalovirus
Congenital viral infection that, in its more severe forms, produces symptoms similar to rubella and may cause hearing loss as well as other abnormalities.

D

Deaf culture
Beliefs, traditions, customs, and attitudes of a subgroup of the deaf population.

Decibel
The unit of measure used to describe the level or magnitude of a sound wave. The logarithm of the ratio between two sound intensities, powers, or sound pressures.

Deformity
A deviation from the normal shape or size of a specific portion of the body.

Degeneration
Decline as in the nature or function from a former or original state.

Dementia
A breakdown or deterioration in cognitive function.

Diagnosis
The process of determining the nature of a disease.

Digital
Numerical representation of a signal especially for use by a computer.

DNA
Deoxyribonucleic acid; molecules that carry genetic information.

E

Earmold Earpiece that is connected to the hearing aid for the purpose of directing sound into the external auditory meatus.

Earphone
A transducer system that converts electrical energy from a signal generator, such as an audiometer, into acoustical energy which is then delivered to the ear.

Educational audiology
A subspecialty in audiology that focuses on providing audiologic services in the schools.

Educational Audiology Association (EAA)
Professional organization for audiologists interested in the provision of audiologic services in the schools.

Effusion
Collection of fluid in the middle ear.

Electroacoustic
Refers to the conversion of acoustic energy to electrical energy, or vice versa, for the purpose of sound generation or measurement.

Electromagnetic field
Field of energy produced by electrical current flowing through a coil or wire.

Emission
Acoustic emissions originating in the cochlea and recorded in the ear canal.

Endogenous
Hereditary forms of hearing impairment; literally means, "within the genes."

Endolymph
The fluid contained within the membranous labyrinth of the inner, including the scala media of the cochlea.

Endolymphatic hydrops
Ménière's disease; build up of endolmyph within the cochlea and vestibular labrynth; typical audiologic findings include vertigo, fullness, and fluctuating sensorineural hearing loss.

ENT
Ear, nose, and throat.

Epidemiology
Branch of medical science that deals with incidence, distribution, and control of disease in a population.

Epithelium
Tissue which forms the surfaces of the body.

Etiology
Pertaining to the cause of a disorder or condition.

Exudate discharge
Usually refers to the secretion of fluid from the mucosal lining of the middle ear.

Exogenous
Acquired forms of hearing impairment; literally means "outside the genes."

F

FAAA
Fellow of the American Academy of Audiology.

Fetal alcohol syndrome
Birth defects that may include facial abnormalities, growth deficiency, mental retardation, and other impairments; caused by the mother's abuse of alcohol during pregnancy.

Filter
Pertains to a device that rejects auditory signals at some frequencies while allowing signals at other frequencies to pass.

Fistula
A tubular passage way or duct formed by disease, surgery, injury, or congenital defect; usually connects two organs.

Flaccid
Weakness—such as a flaccid tympanic membrane.

FM
Frequency modulation.

Formant frequencies
Regions of prominent energy distribution in a speech sound associated with resonances of the vocal tract.

Frequency
The number of complete cycles per second for a vibrating system or other repetitive motion. Expressed in units of hertz (Hz).

Frequency response
The output characteristics of hearing aids or other systems as a function of frequency.

Functional hearing loss
Audiometric evidence of hearing loss when there is no organic basis to explain the hearing loss.

Fundamental frequency
The harmonic component of a complex wave that has the lowest frequency and commonly the greatest amplitude.

G

Gain
For hearing aids, the difference in dB between the input level of an acoustic signal and the output level.

Gene
The biologic unit of heredity, self-reproducing and located in a definite position on a particular chromosome.

Genetic
Related to heredity.

Genetic counseling
Providing information to families with regard to the probability of an inherited disorder.

Genetics
The study of heredity.

Genotype
The genetic makeup of an individual.

Geriatric
Related to the aging process.

Gestational age
Time between mother's last menstrual period and time of baby's birth.

H

Habilitation
Provision of intervention services designed to overcome the handicapping conditions associated with congenital hearing loss.

Hair cells
One of the sensory cells in the organ of Corti.

Handicap
Conditions that impact psychosocial function and the consequence of a disability.

Hard of hearing
HOH; residual hearing is sufficient to enable successful processing of linguistic information through audition with the use of amplification.

Harmonic
A component frequency of a complex wave that is an integer multiple of the fundamental frequency.

Hearing aid
A personal electroacoustic device, typically worn in or on the ear of persons with impaired hearing, which primarily serves to amplify sound arriving at the wearer's ear so as to compensate for the wearer's hearing loss.

Hearing aid performance inventory
Communication scale which assesses the impact of hearing loss across several dimensions including speech comprehension, signal intensity, response to auditory failure, social effects of hearing loss, and occupational difficulties.

Hearing handicap inventory for the elderly
Specific self-report communication scale comprised of items dealing with social situational and emotional aspects of hearing loss.

Hearing impairment
A generic term indicating disability that may range from slight to complete deafness.

Hearing loss
A reduction in the ability to perceive sound; may range from slight to complete deafness.

Hearing sensitivity
The ability of the human ear to perceive sound.

Helicotrema
Passage that connects the scala tympani and the scala vestibuli at the apex of the cochlea.

Hereditary
Genetically transmitted or transmittable from parent to offspring.

Hereditary deafness
Genetically transmitted deafness.

Hertz
A unit of frequency equal to one cycle per second.

High-risk register
Conditions for which children are at greater-than-average risk for hearing impairment.

HINT
Hearing in noise test.

Hyperbilirubinemia
An abnormally large amount of bilirubin in the circulating blood.

Hypertelorism
An abnormal increased distance between two organs or parts.

Hypoxia
Depletion of oxygen.

Hz
Hertz.

I

Identification audiometry
Typically refers to methods used to screen for hearing loss in a simple, quick, and cost-effective manner.

Idiopathic
Pertaining to unknown causation.

Immittance
A general term describing measurements made of tympanic membrane impedance, compliance, or admittance.

Impairment
Abnormal or reduced function.

Impedance
Opposition to the flow of energy through a system; reciprocal of admittance.

Incidence
Proportion of a group initially free of a given condition that develops the condition over time.

Inclusion
Integration of hearing-impaired children into a regular classroom setting.

Incus
The middle bone of the three ossicles in the middle ear; anvil.

Individualized education plan (IEP)
Plan developed by a multidisciplinary team for educating children with disabilities including hearing loss; mandated by IDEA 97 and updated on an annual basis.

Individuals with Disabilities Education Act (IDEA)
Legislation which insures that children with disabilities over the age of 3 years receive a free and appropriate education; also encourages services for children under 3 years old.

Inertia
The tendency of a body to remain in its current state (either motion or rest).

Inner ear
The organ of hearing and equilibrium that is located in the temporal bone.

Insertion gain
Real ear measurement of the gain of a hearing aid.

Intensive care unit (ICU)
Pertains to a separate, designated service area in a hospital that is used for the care and treatment of critically ill patients.

Ipsilateral
Typically refers to the same side.

ITC hearing aid
In the canal hearing aid.

ITE hearing aid
In the ear hearing aid.

J

Jaundice
A yellowish pigmentation of the skin, tissues, and body fluids caused by the deposition of bile pigments.

JCIH
Joint Committee on Infant Hearing—organization comprised of several different organizations including, but not limited to, the American Academy of Audiology, the American Academy of Otolaryngology, the American Academy of Pediatrics, and the American Speech-Language-Hearing Association.

JND
Just noticeable difference.

K

Kanamycin
An ototoxic antibiotic substance consisting of two amino sugars.

Kernicterus
A form of jaundice occurring within the newborn; known to be associated with sensorineural hearing loss.

L

Labyrinth
Maze. In hearing, refers to inner ear.

Labyrinthitis
Inflammation of the labyrinth or inner ear.

Language
The code used by members of the same culture or group to decipher or produce sequences of sounds capable of

communicating thoughts, ideas, and actions to other members of the same culture or group.

Larynx
Anatomical structure housing the vocal cords.

Latency
The period of apparent inactivity between the time a stimulus is presented and the moment a response occurs.

Learning disability
Generic term used to denote learning problems in young school-aged children.

Lesion
Wound or injury; area of pathologic change in tissue.

Lexicon
Mental dictionary representing the words known by an individual for a specific language.

Localization
Pertaining to the identification of sound in space (horizontal or vertical plane).

Loudness discomfort level
LDL; the intensity level that causes discomfort for an individual.

M

Malleus
The largest auditory ossicle; sometimes referred to as the hammer.

Mask
Refers to the ability of one acoustic signal to obscure the presence of another acoustic signal so that it cannot be detected.

Ménière's disease
Endolymphatic hydrops disease of the membranous inner ear characterized by progressive or fluctuating sensorineural hearing loss, vertigo (dizziness), tinnitus (ringing in ears), and sometimes a fullness sensation.

Meningitis
Inflammation of the meninges caused by bacterial or viral infections causing severe to profound sensorineural hearing loss in some cases (10%).

Microtia
A term that implies a small deformed pinna (or auricle).

Meniscus
A crescent shaped structure.

Medial
Toward the axis, near the midline.

Microphone
Transducer that converts acoustical energy into electrical energy.

Mixed hearing loss
Type of hearing loss that includes both conductive and sensorineural impairments.

Monaural
Pertaining to one ear.

Montage
Placement configuration of electrodes in electrophysiologic measurements.

Mucus
Viscous secretion of mucous glands.

Mumps
A contagious viral disease occurring mainly in children; symptoms include parotitis, fever, headaches, and sudden profound unilateral sensorineural hearing loss.

Myringitis
Inflammation of the tympanic membrane.

Myelin
The fatty sheath or covering of the axon of a neuron.

Myringotomy
Surgical procedure that involves making an incision in the eardrum to release pressure, remove fluid, and restore hearing sensitivity.

N

Narrow-band noise
Band of noise limited to a restricted frequency region by filtering.

Nasopharynx
The part of the pharynx (throat) behind and above the soft palate, directly continuous with the nasal passages.

Neomycin
An ototoxic antibiotic, administered orally or locally.

Neonate
Young child—usually during the first 4 weeks.

Nephritis
Inflammation of the kidney.

Nephrotoxic
Toxic to the nephrons of the kidney.

Neuron
Any of the conducting cells of the nervous system; a neuron consists of a cell body, containing the nucleus and the surrounding autoplasm, an axon and a dendrite.

Neuritis
Inflammation of a nerve.

Neurologist
An expert in neurology or in treatment of disorders of the nervous system.

Neurology
Branch of medical science which deals with the nervous system, both normal and in disease.

NICU
Neonatal intensive care unit.

NIHL
Noise induced hearing loss.

Noise-induced hearing loss
Permanent sensorineural hearing loss as a result of exposure to high noise levels.

Nonorganic hearing loss
See functional hearing loss.

Northwestern Auditory Test Number 6
Common open set monosyllabic word test used in the audiologic assessment to determine word recognition ability at comfortable listening levels.

O

Occlusion
Blockage or obstruction; typically refers to the ear canal.

Octave
The interval between two sounds with a 2:1 ratio in frequency.

Ohm
Unit of resistance representing opposition to the transference of energy.

Otitis media
Inflammation of the middle ear space.

Otitis media with effusion
OME; denotes inflammation of the middle ear cleft with a collection of fluid.

Opacification
The development of opacity (impervious to light rays), as of the cornea or lens.

Organ of Corti
Sensory organ of hearing located on the basilar membrane.

Ossicles
Refers to the three bones of the middle ear; malleus, incus, and stapes.

Otalgia
Pertaining to the pain in the ear.

Otitis
Inflammation of the ear.

Otitis prone
Refers to individual who has a predisposition for middle ear disease.

OTO
Otolaryngology.

Otoacoustic emission (OAE)
Sounds produced by the cochlea; usually evoked by an auditory stimulus but can occur spontaneously; considered an outer hair cell phenomenon.

Otolaryngologist
Physician who specializes in diseases of the ear, nose, and throat.

Otolaryngology
Medical specialty associated with diagnosis and management of diseases of the ear, nose, and larynx.

Otologist
A physician who specializes in diseases of the ear.

Otorrhea
Discharge from the ear.

Otosclerosis
Formation of spongy bone in the labrynthine capsule and the stapes footplate. The most common site of the formation is just in front of the oval window. The disease produces impaired stapedial mobility and a gradual conductive hearing loss. Sometimes referred to as otospongiosis.

Otoscope
Hand held device for visual inspection of the ear canal and eardrum.

Ototoxic
Pertains to toxic effects to the ear.

Outer ear
Pertaining to the auricle, external auditory meatus, and the lateral portion of the tympanic membrane.

Outer hair cells
OHC; hair cells within the organ of Corti.

P

Pascal
The unit of sound pressure, abbreviated Pa.

PB
Phonetically balanced.

PB Max
Intensity level at which maximum understanding for phonetically balanced words is achieved.

PBK Word List
Word recognition test used with children; words are within the receptive vocabulary of most school-age children.

Pediatric audiologist
Audiologist who specializes in the assessment and management of young children.

Perforation
Small hole; typically refers to perforation of the tympanic membrane.

Perilymph
The fluid contained within the space separating the membranous from the osseous labrynth of the inner ear, including the scala vestibuli and scala tympani of the cochlea.

Perinatal
Pertains to a condition that occurs in the period shortly before or after birth (from 8 weeks before birth to 4 weeks after).

Periosteum
Specialized connective tissue covering all bones of the body, consisting of a dense, fibrous outer layer and a more delicate inner layer capable of forming bone.

Peripheral
Toward the outward surface or port.

Petrous
Denoting or pertaining to the hard, dense portion of the temporal bone containing the internal auditory organs.

Pneumatic otoscope
Hand-held instrument used to examine visually the external acoustic meatus and the tympanic membrane. A pneumatic bulb connected to the otoscope allows the examiner to vary air pressure in the canal while examining the mobility of the eardrum.

Postnatal
A condition acquired later in life.

Potential
Electric tension or pressure; electric activity in a muscle or nerve cell during activity.

Prenatal
Something that occurs to the fetus before birth.

Presbycusis
Hearing loss due to the aging process.

Prevalence
The number of cases of hearing impairment in a given population at a given point in time.

Psychogenic hearing loss
See functional hearing loss.

Pure-tone audiometry
The measurement of hearing thresholds for pure tones of various frequencies

using standardized equipment and procedures.

Pure-tone average
(PTA); average of hearing thresholds at 500 Hz, 1000 Hz, and 2000 Hz.

R

Real-ear aided response
REAR; Real ear measurement, with a probe-tube microphone, of the SPL as a function of frequency with the hearing aid in place and turned on.

Real-ear unaided response
REUR; Real ear measurement, with a probe-tube microphone, of the SPL as a function of frequency in the ear canal without the hearing aid in place.

Real-ear insertion gain
REIG; probe microphone measurement of the difference between the unaided response and the real ear aided response. REIG = REAR – REUR.

Recruitment
Refers to an abnormally fast growth of loudness with increasing sound intensity in an ear with sensorineural hearing loss once threshold has been exceeded.

Recessive Hereditary Sensorineural Hearing Loss
Form of hereditary deafness; both parents of a child with hearing loss are clinically normal—appearance of the trait requires that the individual possess two similar abnormal genes, one from each parent. The recessive genes account for the transmission of hearing loss; can skip several generations.

Reticular lamina
Net-like layer extending over the surface of the organ of Corti.

Reflex
An involuntary, relatively invariable adaptive response to a stimulus.

Rehabilitation
Management strategies used to restore function following insult or injury.

Renal
Term that refers to the kidney.

Residual hearing
Refers to hearing that remains in individuals with hearing impairment.

Resonance
A frequency region for which the maximum transference of energy through a system occurs.

Retinitis
Inflammation of the retina.

Retrocochlear
Refers to beyond the cochlea, especially nerve fibers along the auditory pathways from the internal auditory meatus to the cortex.

Reverberation
Persistence of sound within an enclosed space following its termination.

Rubella
German measles; a mild viral infection characterized by a pinkish rash which occurs first on the face before spread-

ing to other parts of the body. If contracted during pregnancy, especially during the first trimester, abnormalities of the fetus can result producing mental retardation, hearing loss, visual complications, and mild heart problems.

S

SNR Signal-to-noise ratio; usually refers to the relative difference in dB between the signal (usually speech) and (ambient) noise.

Sagittal Plane
A vertical plane through the longitudinal axis dividing the body into left and right portions.

Scala
A subdivision of the cavity of the cochlea.

Scala media
Middle cavity within the cochlea; filled with endolmyph and contains the organ of corti.

Scala tympani
Perilymph filled cavity below the scala media. Includes the round window.

Scala vestibuli
Perilymph filled cavity above the scala media. Includes the oval window.

Screening
A program designed to expediently and reliably identify those likely to have a disorder within the general population. More definitive follow-up testing is typically required to confirm (or refute) the findings of the screening.

Semantics
The meaning(s) associated with the words of a language.

Sensation level
SL; refers to the level of a signal (dB) above one's threshold.

Sensitivity
Proportion of truly hearing impaired persons in a screened population correctly identified by a screening test.

Serous
A clear fluid free of debris and bacteria.

Serous otitis media
Inflammation of the middle ear with a collection of clear, thin fluid.

Sickle cell anemia
Hereditary disease of the blood that occurs predominately in blacks.

SOAE
Spontaneous otoacoustic emission.

Sound-field
An area (usually a room) into which sound is introduced (usually by a loudspeaker).

Sound pressure level
SPL; magnitude of sound relative to a reference pressure (0.00002 pascals).

Sound wave
A disturbance created in a medium, such as air, by a source of vibration.

Specificity
Proportion of truly normal hearing persons in a screened population correctly identified by a screening test.

Speech audiometry
The measurement of speech recognition threshold (SRT) in decibels and measures of the ability to understand speech when it is many decibels above this threshold.

Speech reception threshold
SRT; threshold for speech using spondaic words; the sound level representing the lowest sound level at which speech can be heard 50% of the time.

Speechreading
Also often referred to as "lip reading", this is the process whereby the listener uses the visible facial gestures of the talker (not just the talker's lips) during speech production to better understand the spoken message.

Spectrum
Display of a sound's amplitude (amplitude spectrum) or phase (phase spectrum) as a function of frequency. Plural form is spectra.

Spiral ganglion
Group of nerve cell bodies located in the modiolus of the cochlea, from which nerve fibers extend into the spiral organ.

Spondee
Two syllable words (e.g., baseball, cowboy) spoken with equal stress on each syllable.

Stapes
The innermost ossicle of the middle ear (stirrup).

Stigmata
Findings or landmarks indicative of a specific disorder.

Streptomycin
Ototoxic antibiotic.

Suppurative
Pus or fluid often found in acute otitis media; characterized by white blood cells, cellular debris, and many bacteria.

Symmetrical hearing loss
Hearing loss that is essentially equivalent in both ears.

Synapse
Region of contact between processes of two adjacent neurons where a nervous impulse is transmitted from one neuron to another.

Syndrome
A group of symptoms that are characteristic of a specific condition or disease.

Syntax
The rules of a language used to string words together into meaningful phrases or sentences. The grammar of a language.

T

Tactile Pertaining to touch.

TC
Total communication; intervention approach which incorporates a combination of auditory/oral and manual communication techniques.

Tangible Reinforcement Operant Conditioning Audiometry
TROCA; reinforcement technique for difficult to test children; child receives reinforcement (candy, cereal, toys) for the correct identification of a signal.

Tectorial membrane
Membrane which projects like a roof over the organ of Corti; the edge of the outer hair cells are embedded within the tectorial membrane.

Temporary threshold shift (TTS)
Temporary elevation of an auditory threshold after exposure to noise. Frequently used to predict the potential danger of a noise environment.

TEOAE
Transient evoked otoacoustic emission; echo emitted by the cochlea in response to a transient stimulus (e.g., click).

Threshold
Softest level at which a stimulus or change in a stimulus can be detected.

Time compression
Process whereby speech is recorded and then played back in less time than the original recording; commonly expressed as a percentage. For example, speech that originally was recorded in 1 second and played back in 1/2 second would be 50% time-compressed.

Tinnitus
Sensation of ringing in the ear.

TM
Tympanic membrane.

Tonotopic
The orderly mapping of sound frequency to anatomical place or location in the auditory system, beginning in the cochlea and proceeding through the auditory portions of the cortex.

TORCH
Acronym used to categorize major infections that may be contracted in utero; Toxoplasmosis, Other, Rubella, Cytomegalovirus, and Herpes simplex. Syphilis has been added to the list to form the acronym STORCH.

Total communication
A manual communication system that is taught to supplement, to varying degrees, the auditory-oral communication of the person with impaired hearing.

Toxoplasmosis
Organism that is transmitted to the child via the placenta. Infection is typically contracted by eating uncooked meat or making contact with the feces of cats. Possible cause of hearing loss.

Transducer
A device or system that converts one form or energy to another.

Tympanogram
Graphic representation of middle ear immittance as a function of air pressure presented to the ear canal.

U

Uncomfortable loudness level
Level (in dB) at which audio signals (pure tones, noise, or speech) become uncomfortably loud.

Unilateral
Refers to one side as in unilateral hearing loss.

Utero
Pertaining to the uterus; the womb.

V

Vibrotactile
Denotes the detection of vibrations via touch.

Vertigo
Dizziness; an illusionary sensation of movement such as spinning or whirling.

Viscosity
The property of fluid which resists change in the shape or arrangement of its element during flow.

Visual Reinforcement Audiometry
VRA; audiologic technique for testing the hearing of young children; a head turn in response to an auditory stimulus is rewarded with a flashing lighted toy or a computerized animated character (e.g., Sponge Bob).

Vocal cords
Cartilaginous structures within the larynx that vibrate when air from the lungs is forced through them. The vibration of the vocal cords is the primary determiner of the pitch of a talker's voice.

Vocal tract
The air-filled cavity between the vocal cords and the lips (or nostrils). Changes in the shape of the vocal tract, primarily via movement of the tongue and velum, change the resonant frequencies of the tract and alter the speech sound produced.

W

Waardenburg Syndrome
A group of genetic conditions that can cause hearing loss and changes in coloring (pigmentation) of the hair, skin, and eyes.

Warble tone
Sound characterized by a continuous fluctuation in frequency of predetermined amount both above and below a central frequency.

Waveform
Display of an acoustic (or electrical) signal with amplitude along the y-axis and time along the x-axis.

Word recognition
Ability to recognize (repeat) monosyllabic words spoken by the clinician when presented well above threshold; typically expressed as percent correct.

Index

A

Acoustic codes, for communication, 44, 45v

Acoustic immittance, 133, 134f, 136
  measurement of, 113, 133–135, 134f, 135f
  in middle-ear disease identification, 176–178
  static, 138

Acoustic intensity (I), 30

Acousticoelectrical transducer, 44

Acoustic reflex, 139, 139f

Acoustic reflex threshold, 138–141, 139f
  in conductive hearing loss, 139–140
  in sensorineural hearing loss, 140

Acoustics. *See* Sound; Sound measurement; Sound wave

Acoustic speech signal, 42

Adenoidectomy, for otitis media, 98

Admittance, 133

Adult rehabilitation, 230–235, 233v. *See also* Rehabilitation, of adult

Age-related hearing loss, 79, 107–109, 108f, 154, 236–238

Air conduction hearing loss, 123–124, 125f

Air conduction hearing measurement, 123–124, 125f, 129v–130v

Air conduction thresholds, 123, 125, 125f, 129v–130v

Air particles
  in sound waves, 16–18, 16v, 17f, 24
  vibration of, 17–18, 17f

Alport syndrome, 83t

American Sign Language (ASL), 5

critical period for learning of, 10–11
sender-receiver fluency in, 5–6

Aminoglycosides, hearing loss from, 104, 126, 127f

Amoxicillin, for otitis media, 97

Amoxicillin/clavulanic, for otitis media, 97

Ampicillin, for otitis media, 97

Amplification, classroom, 205–208, 207f, 209v–210v

Amplification devices, 187–202. *See also* Hearing aids

Amplitude (sound wave), 20, 36–37, 36f
  definition of, 20, 23f
  loudness and, 22
  peak, 19f, 20–22, 23, 23f
  peak-to-peak, 19f, 20–22
  root mean square, 19f, 22
  in speech sounds, 43–44, 43f